Access Your Online Resources

Mentoring for Speech and Language Therapists: Unlocking Professional Development Throughout Your Career is accompanied by a number of printable online materials, designed to ensure this resource best supports your professional needs.

Go to https://resourcecentre.routledge.com/speechmark and click on the cover of this book.

Answer the question prompt using your copy of the book to gain access to the online content.

W0113667

Mentoring for Speech and Language Therapists

In this book, Mary Heritage shows how mentoring can have a powerful impact on the speech and language therapist and their professional development. The text sets out the impact of mentoring at each stage of the speech and language therapist's career – students, novices, practitioners, and leaders – and explores how mentoring is distinct from other supportive relationships that are available, such as counselling, coaching line management, and education. The reader is guided through the process of finding a mentor and making the most of the mentoring relationship. The book goes on to outline what makes a good mentor and concludes with a vision and call to action for the profession to embrace mentoring more widely, with a particular focus on creating a more inclusive professional community.

Each section concludes with a space for reflection and action planning to guide the reader through their own journey of understanding how to use mentoring to unlock their own professional development needs.

This resource is relevant for all speech and language therapists: those embarking on a new career in speech and language therapy, those needing guidance at a career crossroads, leaders looking to develop a workforce, and those wishing to diversify their communication skills to support their colleagues.

Mary Heritage is a speech and language therapist with over 35 years' experience of healthcare, and is now Senior Lecturer at the University of Lincoln, UK. She is interested in developing people throughout their career and practices as a coach-mentor, supporting healthcare professionals at every stage.

Professional Development in Speech and Language Therapy

This series centres on the speech and language therapist and provides practical resources to help the professional grow in confidence and learn new skills allowing them to improve their practice.

Often the busy therapist is consumed with their caseload and their own personal development is put on the back burner. This series provides the reader with practical, accessible resources which allow the reader to focus on themselves, rather than their client. Tailored specifically for the Speech and Language Therapist these books are suitable for newly qualified therapists as well as seasoned professionals who want to add more to their toolkit in a specific area.

Reflective Clinical Supervision in Speech and Language Therapy
Strengthening Supervision Skills
Ruth Howes

Mentoring for Speech and Language Therapists
Unlocking Professional Development Throughout Your Career
Mary Heritage

Mentoring for Speech and Language Therapists

Unlocking Professional Development Throughout Your Career

Mary Heritage

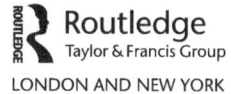

Routledge
Taylor & Francis Group

LONDON AND NEW YORK

Cover image: Getty/Sadeugra

First published 2024
by Routledge
4 Park Square, Milton Park, Abingdon, Oxon OX14 4RN

and by Routledge
605 Third Avenue, New York, NY 10158

Routledge is an imprint of the Taylor & Francis Group, an informa business

© 2024 Mary Heritage

British Library Cataloguing-in-Publication Data
A catalogue record for this book is available from the British Library

ISBN: 978-1-032-47981-1 (hbk)
ISBN: 978-1-032-47980-4 (pbk)
ISBN: 978-1-003-38682-7 (ebk)

DOI: 10.4324/9781003386827

Typeset in Galliard
by Deanta Global Publishing Services, Chennai, India

Contents

Foreword

Many books on mentoring introduce an example as a model of a mentoring relationship taken from a well-known film. Whatever your favourite genre, you will be familiar with a pairing between a mature and wise mentor and our hero, who succeeds, or overcomes, under the guidance of the mentor. There are some excellent examples.

You may be familiar with some of these films and will be able to recall the mentoring conversations:

> Epic fantasies: *Star Wars, Lord of the Rings, The Chronicles of Narnia*
>
> Inspirational teachers of young people: *Harry Potter, Good Will Hunting, Dead Poets Society, Billy Elliott, Mary Poppins*
>
> Sports coaching: *The Karate Kid, Rocky, Coach Carter*
>
> Animation: *Ratatouille, Mulan, The Lion King, Pinocchio*

Before writing a book for a majority female profession, I looked for a female–female pairing, to inspire us from the start. Interestingly, very few examples emerged. My best is from *The Sound of Music* (20th Century Fox, 1965). In the film, Maria has been sent out of the abbey in which she is a novice by the Mother Abbess (her superior) to be a governess to the family of a widower, Captain Von Trapp. Maria returns, unexpectedly, to the abbey to ask Mother Abbess to let her stay and make her final vows.

Watching the scene again, we can identify the younger, less experienced mentee (Maria) and the more mature mentor, Mother Abbess. Maria has initiated the conversation by returning to the abbey. The scene illustrates the structure of a mentoring session between the two:

- Listening: "Tell us what happened."
- Questioning: Mother Abbess poses a series of six questions to prompt Maria, and to gain clarification. Maria responds by narrating the events preceding her return; in doing so, Maria gains a new insight.

Only when Maria says "Please help me" does Mother Abbess have permission to respond. The mentor's offering includes:

- Wisdom: "If you love this man, it doesn't mean you love God less."
- Advice for action: "You must go back."
- Guidance: "These walls were not built to shut out troubles, you have to face them."
- Inspiration: "You have to live the life you are born to live."

Mother Abbess goes on to sing "Climb Ev'ry Mountain", to underline her points.

The scene includes the key elements of a mentoring session (with the exception, maybe, of singing an inspirational number, which I have never experienced – up to this point!)

 References

Wise, R. (dir.) (1965) *The Sound of Music*. Los Angeles: 20th Century Fox.

Introduction

During the second half of my career, I have been struck by the impact of mentors on my development and progress. Looking back, I wonder why mentoring tends not to be talked about within the speech and language therapy profession until we move out of speech and language therapist (SLT) roles and into leadership roles.

Thinking about my early career, my decision to train to become an SLT, and those first steps into the profession, it strikes me as paradoxical that these are the years when mentoring would be most fruitful.

On further reflection, maybe our mentors were always there, but we didn't call them mentors? We called them leaders, managers, supervisors, teachers – and mainly friends. Yet we lose people along the career path, and our profession is crying out for more inclusivity. Did those people have mentors? Or did they have to make a difficult decision alone?

When I set out on this book, I wasn't aware of any literature specifically on mentoring in speech and language therapy. On closer examination, there are important studies from the United States showing that mentoring has a particular benefit to SLTs (or speech and language pathologists in the US), especially in the early career stages – and most especially for those from marginalised groups within the profession.

I became convinced that SLTs have the skill set needed to mentor, and that it is an underutilised resource in our stretched professional community.

DOI: 10.4324/9781003386827-1

This book will help us, as SLTs, to understand what mentoring is and is not. We will look at times in our careers when we could benefit from the support of a mentor, how to find one – and how to get the most out of the relationship. We will then see how we could mentor others along their career journeys, concluding with the impact this could have on our profession.

I intend to challenge the reader – to think about your own mentoring needs, your potential to mentor, and the transformational effect that we could have as a whole profession.

I am indebted to the School of Health and Science at the University of Lincoln, UK for supporting me in this endeavour, and to Victoria Harris, Dr Lindsey Thiel, and David Scoines for time and encouragement. And finally, I acknowledge my own "Wise Owls" and those I am now mentoring for what you have taught me about the subject. Thank you.

What Is Mentoring?

Introduction

According to Greek mythology, the original Mentor (a goddess in disguise) was charged with responsibility for the King's son, Telemachus, and became his wise guide (Rolfe, 2020). The ancient narratives point to a mentor who is one who "counsels, guides, nurtures, advises and enables" (Roberts, 1999). A variant of this meaning developed, more closely related to education and pedagogy, and this was the dominant understanding of mentoring until recent years.

A text about a single topic should start with a working definition. The definitions of mentoring vary according to the point in history and the context. A simple dictionary definition of the mentor is: "a wise or trusted advisor or guide". This points us in a helpful direction.

For a more detailed description, Julie Starr (2014, xi) offers: "A mentor adopts a primarily selfless role in supporting the learning, development and ultimate success of another person."

As for the craft of the mentor: it is a dynamic process that results in the development or learning of the recipient (often referred to as the mentee). Ann Rolfe writes: "Mentoring itself is about evolution – learning, advancement, and personal and professional growth. It is for those who proactively develop themselves" (Rolfe, 2020, viii).

Mentoring is frequently referred to in the context of the development and learning of healthcare professionals. For example, Gopee's (2011) specific definition in the nursing context is: "a formal role in nurse education to direct focus on enabling students to gain safe and

DOI: 10.4324/9781003386827-2

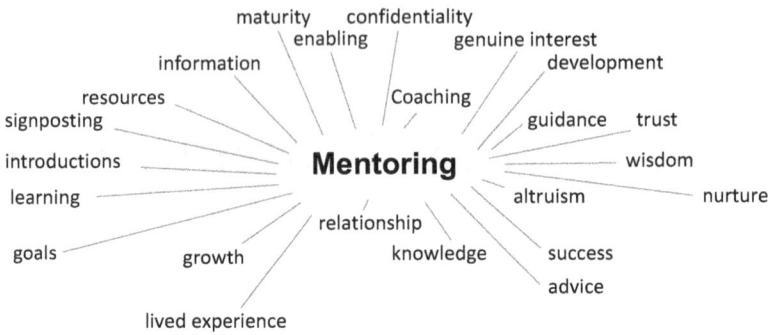

Figure 1.1 The multiple aspects of definitions of mentoring

effective clinical practice skills during practice placements". Most of the literature relating to mentoring healthcare professionals uses this context. However, in speech and language therapy, the enabling of students to develop clinical skills in practice placements is undertaken by the practice educator, so the term "mentoring" has not been used widely.

The multiple aspects of varied definitions of mentoring are shown in Figure 1.1. The key characteristics of mentoring that distinguish it from other supportive relationships are:

- maturity or experience

- altruism (selflessness)

- interest, or investment, in the development of another person

What Is the Evidence for Mentoring?

Eby et al. (2008) undertook a multidisciplinary meta-analysis to assess the impact of mentoring relationships. Compared with those without a mentor, those who had participated in mentoring relationships experienced more positive outcomes in terms of career development, higher job satisfaction and salaries, faster career progression, and psychosocial wellbeing. Subjects with mentors reported higher levels of self-esteem, self-efficacy, confidence, and resilience. The positive impact of mentoring was consistent across different fields and contexts, including both educational and workplace settings.

The evidence base for mentoring specifically within the speech and language therapy profession is limited. We will explore this in Chapter 2.

As there is a lack of a conclusive definition or evidence base for mentoring in the context of the speech and language therapy profession, it may be helpful to consider what mentoring is *not*.

Mentoring shares some characteristics with each of the following, but is not:

- coaching
- counselling
- line management
- leadership
- practice education
- clinical supervision
- mentorship – as used in the context of clinical placement
- preceptorship
- personal tutoring
- advice and guidance services
- friendship

We will now establish how mentoring differs from each of these "talking-based" sources of support.

Coaching

Coaching is a specific non-directive conversation in which a person has protected time to think about a question and find their own way forward. The skill of the coach lies in deep, empathic listening, and in asking carefully crafted questions that challenge or encourage the thinking of the person. The coach may also make observations that enhance the person's insight. Coaching is a person-centred practice based on Carl Rogers' humanistic approach. Peltier describes Rogers' influence on the development of coaching practice in terms of his: "deep faith in the tendency of people to develop in a positive and constructive manner if a climate of respect and trust is established" (Peltier, 2010, 104). Typically, a coach engages with a person for a contracted episode (for example, a series of six coaching sessions), focusing on a particular goal, or set of goals. This could be success in securing a new role, acquiring a new skill, developing resilience, or recovery from an adverse event or episode, for example. Most mentors will adopt a coaching approach to facilitate the person's development. The key difference is that a person will identify their mentor specifically to access the benefit of the mentor's relevant experience. For that reason, the mentor is likely to offer advice, resourced by that experience. So the process may look very similar to the observer, but the selection of the mentor for their experience and the coach for their skill is a nuanced distinction.

Starr (2014) refers to a continuum of coaching and mentoring. In my own coaching practice, I may ask the person for permission to disclose my own experience, or to offer a suggestion. Similarly, I would also draw on my coaching skills while mentoring. The overlap between the roles of coach and mentor has been described as a single skill set: that of "coach-mentor". Bruce-Foulds et al. support this flexibility between the two disciplines: "the most effective approach uses a blend of coaching and mentoring stances, depending on what the client needs – and practitioners who do this are often referred to as coach-mentors" (Bruce-Foulds et al., 2017, 228).

Counselling

Counselling is a talking therapy, and the term covers a wide range of psychodynamic approaches. Counsellors (therapists or psychotherapists) are trained to help the person develop a better understanding of themself and others, usually in relation to a specific emotional issue. This may involve helping them to identify a root cause in the person's past. Counselling may be offered in the context of healthcare provision, related to physical or mental ill health. Like coaching, the skilled counsellor is effective through empathic listening with careful observations and questioning. Unlike mentoring, the counsellor would not be selected for their specific relevant experience of the person's current challenge. In the same way that all healthcare professionals maintain professional boundaries, counsellors cannot become personally invested in the development of the person over time. A mentor is invested in the person's achievements, and therefore lacks the same detached objectivity that counsellors maintain in relation to their clients. The literal meaning of "counsel" is advice (or to advise) – for example, in the context of the legal system. However, counsellors as therapists are more likely to support the person to find their own insight and way forward than to provide advice to them.

Line Management

An employee's line manager is in a position of seniority immediately above them in an organisational hierarchy, and as such has responsibility for their day-to-day performance. Managers are responsible for activities such as operational planning, delivering on organisational goals, recruiting staff, and maximising performance in teams. Managers are engaged in the same business as their staff, therefore the line management role is specific to the occupational context in which the person works. Line managers should also be leaders, developing behaviours and a demeanour that inspire followership. Effective line managers are increasingly encouraged to develop coaching and mentoring skills to effect transformational change in their teams. A line manager is invested in the development of a person, to enhance their contribution to organisational goals as much as to enable them to flourish as an individual. The interest of the manager is therefore not primarily altruistic, unlike the mentor or coach. It is not essential for a manager to have additional skills in developing the individual through conversation – although nowadays, it is more common for organisations to encourage the development of coaching and mentoring approaches in leadership and management.

Leadership

Independent of a formal position or seniority in an organisation, leadership is how one person inspires and enables change in, or through, others. According to Kevin Kruse (2013), "leadership is a process of social influence, which maximises the efforts of others, towards the achievement of a goal". Speech and language therapist Carrie Biddle writes: "The cornerstones of leadership include the ability to build relationships and effectively, and the aptitude to guide others to a better future place with positive impact, and in such a way that people choose to engage and follow" (Biddle, 2020, 11). In contemporary society and workplaces, all individuals, regardless of position or rank, are encouraged to develop and exhibit leadership acumen. At all stages of our careers, we can take steps that will lead to transformational change. Leadership is therefore very different from coaching, counselling, or managing – all of which develop through qualification or appointment. Like mentoring, leadership is a set of skills developed by the individual, and a person identifies someone that they regard as a mentor or leader within their own sphere. Any leader is equipped to mentor others. The ability to inspire followership is a skill set that would equip them to mentor others through a trusting relationship: experience or expertise and an authentic interest in developing others are the hallmarks of mentorship. We will return to the expansion of mentoring in our profession in Chapter 6.

Clinical Supervision

Clinical supervision is a process specific to healthcare. It originated in mental health, psychology, and nursing. There is now a common expectation for health professionals to contribute to their ongoing registration. It refers to a relationship between two or more clinically focused peers:

> *The clinical supervisor undergoes educational preparation for this role and utilises clinical knowledge and experience to assist peers to further develop their own knowledge, competence, values and practices.*
>
> (Gopee, 2011, 14)

Speech and language therapists (SLTs) are required by the regulator, the Health and Care Professions Council (HCPC), to "work in partnership with colleagues, sharing your skills, knowledge, and experience where appropriate, for the benefit of service users and carers" (HCPC, 2016, Standard 2.5). Clinical supervision is one important way in which registrants can fulfil this requirement. As in mentoring, the clinical supervisor is required to have experience in a relevant clinical skill or practice and, to some extent, will invest in the person's development. Unlike mentoring, the supervisor generally shares the same profession, specialism, and organisation as the supervisee, although that is not always the case. In specialist roles, we may seek a clinical supervisor from outside our immediate team or employing organisation. Speech and language therapists working outside clinical practice access other types of supervision – for example, research supervision.

Practice Education

Speech and language therapy students undertaking a pre-registration programme in the United Kingdom are required by the professional body and by the regulator to undertake a minimum of 150 sessions of practice-based learning (Royal College of Speech and Language Therapists [RCSLT], 2021). This provides the opportunity to consolidate academic learning, apply their learning, and develop their clinical and professional skills in the practice setting.

The RCSLT stipulates: "Practising SLTs are required to provide excellent clinical learning opportunities to support, inspire and enable them to serve our clients in the best way they can, and to future-proof our profession" (RCSLT, 2021). It is the role of the practice educator to provide those learning experiences. The skills of the practice educator include signposting information, sharing experience, and coaching. There is an investment in the development of the student. In these ways, a practice educator has similarities with a mentor. The role is not, however, voluntary. The student does not select their practice educator. There is a third-party relationship, in that the practice educator is accountable to the university for the quality and quantity of practice learning, and for providing feedback and the ultimate outcome for the student on their placement. The practice educator ultimately has to give the student a grade that will impact the outcome of the placement, and therefore there is a power imbalance.

Mentorship (in Relation to Clinical Placements)

While practice-based learning for speech and language therapists takes place under the supervision of a practice educator, in nurse education the role is fulfilled by a mentor. As defined by the Nursing and Midwifery Council (2008), the mentor "facilitates learning and supervises and assesses students in practice settings". This use of the same terminology is included in this chapter to make the distinction, highlighting the risk of confusion when used in interprofessional contexts. The role provided by the nurse mentor is usually referred to as *mentorship*, whereas in this book, for additional clarity, I will use the term *mentoring*.

Personal Tutoring

Alongside the practice educator, the personal tutor is a member of the academic team who provides a complementary function in the student's professional development: "One who improves the intellectual and academic ability, and nurtures the emotional wellbeing of learners through individualised, holistic support" (Stork and Walker, 2015, 3). Like a mentor, the personal tutor has a particular interest in the personal welfare of each tutee, and their achievements. Like the practice educator, the tutor is allocated to the student, not selected, and is accountable to the university, and so differs from a mentor. During the student's pre-registration learning, the personal tutor may fulfil the function of a mentor. The personal tutor would also be approached to provide a reference to the student's employer or another university following graduation, but is unlikely to mentor ex-students after completing their qualification.

Preceptorship

Following graduation, and on successful registration with the Health and Care Professions Council, a student embarks on a period of transition from learner to newly qualified practitioner. As a newly autonomous professional, a period of support (usually between four and 12 months) from the employer can offer great value. During the preceptorship period, employers of newly qualified practitioners (NQPs) are encouraged to provide additional support and protected development time. Preceptees are encouraged to identify a designated mentor. Kramer (1974) described the "reality shock" of newly qualified nurses making the transition to autonomous professionals, and their associated attrition. The role of preceptor subsequently became established in the nursing profession. Preceptorship in speech and language therapy is a newer concept – or at least the term has been adopted in our profession more recently. The RCSLT continues to recommend that NQPs secure a buddy, a supervisor, and a mentor. Coordinated preceptorship offers of NHS employers are now more accessible to speech and language therapists and other allied health professionals. According to NHS England (Cox and Wray, 2022), the preceptor should be at the same or a more senior level and a registered healthcare professional within the same discipline, with a minimum of 12 months' experience post-registration. The Department of Health guidance (2010) outlined 12 attributes of an effective preceptor. These share attributes with mentors: a role model, experience, signposting, listening, and facilitating. Like practice educators, line managers and personal tutors, preceptors are not objective, but are accountable to the employing organisation and are likely to be allocated to the NQP, and not selected by them. NHS England currently recommends formal preceptorship at transition points – not only from university to employment as a registered health professional, but also, for example, in transition from one sector or country to another, or returning to practice after a break (NHS England). In its latest guidance on preceptorship, HCPC (2023) reiterates the importance of mentoring for new or returning registrants, and distinguishes preceptorship and mentoring.

Advice and Guidance

For completeness, a speech and language therapist may seek information and direction from a range of Advice and Guidance services. These could be online, or provided by the employer, university, or by a membership organisation (for example, the Royal College of Speech and Language Therapists, the Association of Speech and Language Therapists in Independent Practice, or a trade union), and may provide support with a range of issues: personal, health, career, financial, legal, or welfare. The advantage of an advice and guidance service would be to access timely information, while the benefit of mentoring would be an ongoing relationship with someone with a personal interest in investing in the mentee over an extended period.

Friends and Peers

Many of us initially turn to the people closest to us – trusted friends, colleagues, and family members – for support and guidance. Their role can be the most impactful of all – they have our best interests at heart, and their relationship with us is long term. However, they may not have sufficient breadth of insight into the professional context. We will return to the role of peers across the span of our careers in Chapter 6.

Figure 1.2 shows how all of the above compare with mentoring in terms of their objectivity and context-specificity. Mentoring spans both axes, i.e. it can be objective or involved; specific to or independent of the person's current context.

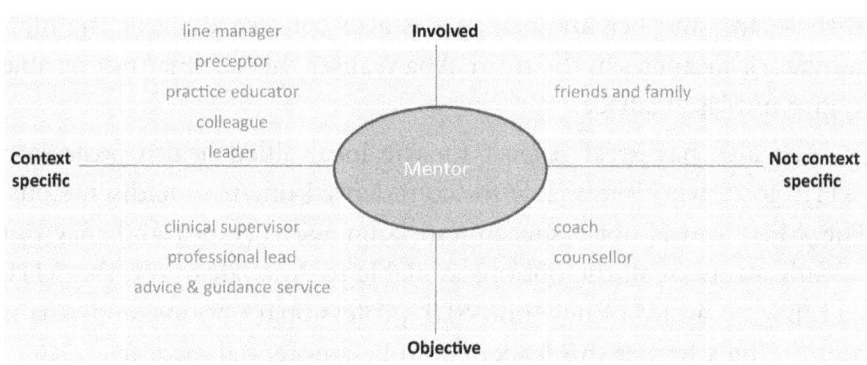

Figure 1.2 Mentoring versus other sources of support

Ana's Story (Part 1)

Ana is a speech and language therapist employed by an NHS hospital Trust. She was involved in an adverse incident that resulted in an investigation, and this has left her questioning her future career direction. As she moves forward from the damaging impact of her recent experience, she is considering what her various options might be.

She recognises that her current feelings have triggered an emotional response echoing those she experienced in her teens. At that point, she felt she couldn't match up to high parental expectations. She wonders whether she could access the wellbeing services provided by her Trust or some counselling through her GP practice. She is motivated to explore the impact of her early experiences on her current identity as a speech and language therapist.

Having lost some confidence in her clinical competence, Ana is already working with her clinical supervisor to explore how she feels, what she's learned, and how she might use appropriate training within the organisation to rebuild her confidence and competence. In the meantime, she will request changes to her caseload and additional support from a more senior colleague via her team leader.

Ana gets on well with her line manager and prepares to raise a question with her about her future direction during her annual performance review – under the section called "Future Career Aspirations for the Next 3 Years". However, she is mindful of staffing shortages in the team, and her line manager is also concerned about the high number of vacancies in the team. Ana realises that she may not be able to give unbiased advice.

Ana also has great respect for the local allied health profession (AHP) lead, who is available for confidential one-to-one discussions. The AHP lead is not a speech and language therapist and may not be fully aware of all the options available to Ana. However, the AHP lead may be aware of new non-SLT professional options, and Ana is considering whether this leader could be a potential mentor.

Ana has also come across an SLT, Kim, who is in a similar AHP leadership role, but in a different county. Ana isn't sure whether she is allowed to ask for help outside her own area, or whether she should stick to the local system.

Ana will talk all of this through with her partner Alex. She is mindful that Alex is anxious about rising costs and job security for them both. She wonders whether the conversation may intensify Alex's concerns that Ana could put herself out of work, and she will be careful about how she raises possible new directions.

Ana remembers Sam, her first practice educator, who has moved into independent practice and is no longer working in the same clinical field. They've kept in touch informally, and she knows Sam's door is open for confidential, unbiased guidance. They met up for a drink when Ana first took on her current role after leaving university. Ana could approach Sam, although Sam may not be up to date on NHS opportunities.

With some searching, Ana discovers that the Trust has a network of coaches, and access to a regional network which advertises a free service to help her find her own answers to her current issues. With three to six online sessions she could find her answers to questions like: "How can I find out if I really want to continue to be an SLT?" and "How can I find someone who can guide me towards new career options that I don't yet know about?"

Ana finds herself with a list of people whom she knows, respects, and could approach. Each of them has a slightly different perspective: they have different views on Ana, and different expectations of her – and each has a unique understanding of the world in which Ana is finding her next steps. She wonders whether to talk to all of them – this would be time-consuming and potentially confusing, but would have the benefit of drawing from all their wisdom. On the other hand, this may not be a one-off conversation, and the idea of an ongoing relationship with someone to advise and guide her is appealing. She lists pros and cons against each of their names.

In the chapters to come, we will follow Ana as she identifies and approaches a potential mentor.

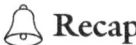 Recap

A **mentor** is a "a wise or trusted advisor or guide".

Mentoring someone involves:

- maturity or experience

- altruism (selflessness)

- interest in the development of another person

The mentor may be experienced in the same or a related context, and the mentor may or may not offer objectivity.

Mentoring is not the same as coaching, counselling, line management, leadership, clinical supervision, practice education, personal tutoring, preceptorship, and friendship. There are both similarities and distinctions between mentoring and each of them.

Reflection Prompts

You may find it helpful to pause now to reflect on and note:

- What is the question that I'm looking to find an answer to?

- Who is available to me through my employer?

- What value would someone with more objectivity offer? What about someone from a different context?

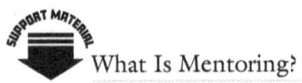

▦ Action Plan

My next step could involve sharing my thoughts with:			
	✓	✗	?
Someone close to me: • family • someone I studied with			
Someone with insight into my context • colleague • line manager • other leader			
Early career only: • practice educator • preceptor			
Someone less closely involved: • clinical supervisor • professional lead			
Someone with complete objectivity: • coach • counsellor			
Someone not directly involved but with relevant experience or insight: • mentor • advice service			

Further Reading

Part 1, "Mentoring Defined", in Ann Rolfe's *Mentoring Mindset, Skills, and Tools* (2020)

Chapter 1, "What Is Mentoring? And What Is It Not?", in Julie Starr's *The Mentoring Manual* (2014)

References

Biddle, C. (2020) Living leadership. *Royal College of Speech and Language Therapists Bulletin*, 11 (March). Available from: https://www.rcslt.org/wp-content/uploads/media/Project/Bulletins/bulletin-2020/march-bulletin-2020.pdf#page=11.

Bruce-Foulds, C., Clark, G. and Ray, K. (2017) In Parsloe, E. and Leedham, M. (Eds.), *Coaching and Mentoring: What Are They and How Are They Used in Organisations?*. London: Kagan Page, 225–242.

Cox, D. and Wray, J. (2022) National preceptorship framework for nursing. Available from: https://www.england.nhs.uk/long-read/national-preceptorship-framework-for-nursing/ [accessed on 13/12/2022].

Department of Health (2010a) Preceptorship framework for newly registered nurses, midwives and allied health professionals. In Gopee, N. (Ed.), *Mentoring and Supervision in Healthcare*. London: SAGE. https://cddft.nhs.uk/media/238368/preceptorship%20framework.pdf

Eby, L. T., Allen, T. D., Evans, S. C., Ng, T. and DuBois, D. L. (2008) Does mentoring matter? A multidisciplinary meta-analysis comparing mentored and non-mentored individuals. *Journal of Vocational Behavior*, 72 (2), 254–267.

Gopee, N. (2011) *Mentoring and Supervision in Healthcare* (2nd edition). London: SAGE.

Health and Care Professions Council (2016) *Standards of Conduct, Performance and Ethics*. London: Standard 2.5 [accessed 13/12/2022].

Health and Care Professions Council (2023) *Principles for Preceptorship – Helping Health and Care Professionals through Career Transitions*. London [accessed 4/3/2024].

Kramer, M. (1974) Reality shock: Why nurses leave nursing. *American Journal of Nursing*, 75 (5), 891.

Kruse, K. (2013) What is leadership? *Forbes*. Available from: https://www.forbes.com/sites/kevinkruse/2013/04/09/what-is-leadership/?sh=477089e95b90 [accessed on 13/12/2022].

NHS England. Available from: https://www.hee.nhs.uk/our-work/allied-health-professions/education-employment/national-allied-health-professionals-preceptorship-foundation-support-programme/preceptorship [accessed on 3/10/2023].

Nursing and Midwifery Council (2008) *A Standard to Support Learning and Assessment in Practice*. London: NMC.

Peltier, B. (2010) *The Psychology of Executive Coaching, Theory and Application* (2nd edition). New York: Routledge.

RCSLT (2021) Practice based learning guidance: Key requirements. Available from: https://www.rcslt.org/members/lifelong-learning/practice-based-learning/practice-based-learning-guidance-introduction/#section-6 [accessed on 3/10/2023].

Roberts, A. (1999) The origins of the term mentor. *History of Education Society Bulletin*, 64 (November), 313–329.

Rolfe, A. (2020) *Mentoring Mindset, Skills, and Tools* (4th edition). South West Rocks, NSW: Mentoring Works.

Starr, J. (2014) *The Mentoring Manual*. Harlow: Pearson Education Limited.

Stork, A. and Walker, B. (2015) *Becoming an Outstanding Personal Tutor; Supporting Learners through Personal Tutoring and Coaching*. Northwich: Critical Publishing.

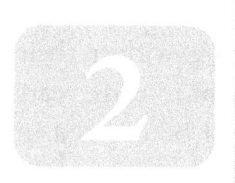

Mentoring in Speech and Language Therapy

This chapter will identify where mentoring can support the development of a speech and language therapist (SLT) during their career, and will suggest potential roles for mentors to resource SLTs at every stage of their career for the purposes of:

- continuing professional development
- resilience and wellbeing
- leadership development
- pre-registration learning
- preceptorship
- career progression through to retirement

Introduction

A review of the available literature to establish what evidence exists to inform our understanding of mentoring in the context of the speech and language therapy profession, identified the following areas of published work:

- mentoring for allied health professions, generally (McPherson et al., 2006; Mak et al., 2022) or specifically (e.g., physiotherapy: Buning and Buning, 2019; Naidoo et al., 2021), provides insights that may have relevance for the speech and language therapy profession

DOI: 10.4324/9781003386827-3

- mentoring for diversity (Rodriguez, 2016), which will be covered in Chapter 5: Atherton, Davidson, and McAllister (2017)

- the skills needed by SLTs to provide mentoring within their clinical practice (e.g., supporting staff development in early years settings: Kent and McDonald, 2021), which will be covered in Chapter 4

The published literature that specifically focuses on mentoring within the speech and language therapy profession explores either the benefits for the professional and their own development or the value for the people they support (their patients or service users). Most of this evidence base, originates from the United States. The US professional body for speech and language pathology (SLP), the American Speech and Hearing Association (ASHA), warrants mention for its innovative "Gathering Place" and "Student to Empowered Professional" (STEP) initiatives. Gathering Place was established in 2004, bringing together speech and language therapy professionals and students, including PhD students (Burger, 2009; Tucker, 2013; ASHA, 2012; Lewis, 2015). There is a particular emphasis on the value of mentoring for therapists from communities which are currently underrepresented in the profession (which will be explored further in Chapter 5) and on early-stage professionals (pre-registration students, newly qualified SLTs and preceptees).

My experience suggests that SLTs are more likely to identify a mentor when they are seeking career advancement beyond the SLT role. For example, in my own career, I thought about finding a mentor when I left my SLT management role and took up a senior leadership position which included allied health profession (AHP) leadership responsibilities for the organisation. Maybe we believe that within the SLT profession we have adequate sources of support, but that outside our professional world an independent guide would be helpful? Alternatively, maybe mentors are now a recognised source of support for leaders in senior positions. SLTs progressing their careers into higher management may be signposted to finding a mentor when they reach this point in their career.

This chapter will look first at the benefits of mentoring in early careers, and then at mentoring to support ongoing continuing professional development (CPD) and career development throughout the SLT's career.

Early Careers/Pre-registration Learning/Career Choice

Career Selection

Before looking at how a mentor could enrich the early career development of SLTs, the question arose as to how soon a speech and language therapy student should identify a mentor. Surely there are few career crossroads more significant than the point of career choice. As Programme Lead for a master's pre-registration programme, I am regularly approached by graduates who are seeking information about the programme. My advice is always to check that they are sufficiently informed about the career path they have chosen before they commit to an intensive and personally demanding period of study. I've also observed that applicants often refer to members of the profession who have generously shared their time and advice at this stage. Now that there are multiple routes to registration – bachelor's, master's, apprenticeship, full- or part-time, for example, as well as the choice of local or more distant universities – a member of the profession, carefully selected, could help would-be students make a wise decision from the outset.

Competition for pre-registration training places at UK universities is high. The cost – personally and financially – to students who leave the course without completing it is also unacceptable. Health Education England's RePAIR (2018) project reported on a survey of students in nursing, midwifery, and therapeutic radiography and makes a recommendation to help students "understand in advance of starting their course, the challenges and demands of their chosen career and study".

There is no better time to identify a mentor within the profession to support and guide the next generation of SLTs through their decision making. This could result in future student cohorts being sufficiently informed to make a commitment to enter the profession, and to complete the course successfully. There is a role for university tutors in the profession to suggest this as a first step, or to identify it as a positive indicator in personal statements and at interview. It could also be recommended preparation for offer-holders before they enrol at the start of their studies. However, this would disadvantage those who do not have friends and family working within health and social care, who would find it much harder to identify a suitable mentor. An opportunity presents itself to the profession, and to universities, to support all students to find an early career mentor, with a particular emphasis on those who lack the privilege of friends and family networks.

Enquirers seeking mentorship at this stage might look for:

- an informed SLT with recent or current exposure to routes to registration

- open-mindedness

- listening and coaching skills

- asking carefully crafted questions to elicit the motivations and priorities of the enquirer

- knowledge of the current demands of pre-registration education – e.g., funding opportunities, curricula

- knowledge of employment opportunities across the profession and/or in a given region

- access to Royal College of Speech and Language Therapists (RCSLT) careers resources

SLTs who are approached by someone making their career choice might consider their skills in relation to those listed above and their ability to offer some support by:

- asking more questions in preference to giving opinions or advice

- finding out about the enquirer (hearing their story)

- signposting to resources (e.g., the RCSLT, the Health and Care Professions Council [HCPC])

- signposting to online resources about people who benefit from speech and language therapy services – these might be online communities, feature films, documentaries, books, social media accounts, or podcasts

- signposting to work or voluntary experience that broadens the enquirer's understanding – not only of the profession, but perhaps more importantly, of people with special communication and eating, drinking, and swallowing needs

- signposting to career decision making resources (e.g., *The Career Coach* by Corinne Mills, 2007)

- creating a space in which the enquirer can think (see Nancy Kline's work, e.g., *Time to Think*, 1998)

One example of good practice came from an experienced SLT who mentors undergraduate students with an interest in pursuing a career in speech and language therapy:

I wear several "hats" as a mentor: describing what the role of a Speech and Language Therapist is (and is not), which universities offer training and the differences between these, the process of applying for a course, the role of the Royal College of Speech and Language Therapists and the Health and Care Professions Council, what volunteer opportunities there are that may support a course application and of course, sharing my clinical experiences, successes, challenges and "kodak" moments! My role is to hold a space where not only can I inspire, enthuse, and motivate students to want to enter the profession but where students feel comfortable to ask questions and clarify information about the role – after all, this is their future they are planning! Sometimes it's a one-off conversation to give information and sometimes it's support with applications and keep in touch throughout the course. It's always led by the mentee. I'm available if they need me.

(Brown, 2023)

Pre-registration Learning

At first glance, we might think that students in pre-registration training are well supported in their professional development. As they lay their career foundations, they benefit from the input of their lecturers, personal tutor, university careers service, practice educators, and peers to meet most of their needs. Pre-registration programmes integrate learning opportunities from academic study (teaching and assessments) and practice education (placements). So it may not be initially evident what is the added value of yet another supporter at this point. Yet this is also perhaps the most demanding stage of the SLT's career. Most professionals reach a point in their training where they struggle to continue, maybe comparable to a runner "hitting the wall" during a marathon. Maybe this is the point when a mentor could add great value – someone with objectivity who is invested in the development of the "novice" speech and language therapist (borrowing a nursing term from Benner, 1982).

In a study by Quigley et al. (2020), students were surveyed as they made the transition from classroom to more dynamic placement learning. The findings of this study conclude that the optimal learning environment for practice education (placements) includes mentoring, supervision, and feedback – all fulfilled by the practice educator.

Some studies have explored this further.

Matthews et al. (2021), working in a US university, at the graduate school level (which equates to postgraduate pre-registration education in the UK), reported on a peer mentoring scheme to support graduates moving into master's-level study. They described the challenges students face in a competitive admissions process. "Peer mentoring" is one initiative offered to equip those graduates to be successful in their applications for graduate school.

Citing Kent (2006), Matthews et al. hypothesised that there would be mutual benefits for the mentee and mentor in terms of "increased career satisfaction, productivity and the sharing of ideas"

(Matthews et al., 2021). Students were randomly allocated a mentor, and each mentor was assigned four or five more junior students to mentor for a minimum of one month. If this model were applied to a UK university department, final-year students might mentor first-year students. Their conclusions were that mentoring developed "collaborative learning and relationships" within the learning community and were part of the way the university enabled students to compete within the graduate admissions process.

Two previous studies, Saenz (2000) and Wright-Harp and Cole (2008), reported increased student retention within communication sciences and disorders (equivalent to speech and language therapy pre-registration programmes in the UK) when students have mentors.

In a separate study, Greene (2021) found that second-year SLP mentors may have had a positive impact on the perceived stress levels of their first-year mentees. Barbara Conrad, looking back on a 26-year career as an SLP, provides a personal view of the contribution of two SLP friends whose support and encouragement was sustained throughout her career. In turn, she reflected, she went on to connect 25 students with "home-team" mentors who encouraged the students through their courses:

> *I recognize many who were influential in my career, but two people played key roles in my career development. They were friends – who can be the best mentors! I highly encourage anyone starting out, changing jobs, or feeling in a "slump" to phone a friend.*
>
> (Conrad, 2006, 57)

STEP offers a condensed mentoring programme that supports students to achieve a development goal for students from racial or ethnic minority backgrounds (ASHA, 2012). This article goes on to say that the STEP programme is open to all students, but those from minority communities are given preference.

A similar scheme has been developed in the UK at Leeds Beckett University, under the leadership of Dr Lindsey Thiel. This mentor scheme matches speech and language therapists from groups that are under-represented within the profession with any speech and language therapy students at the university who would like a mentor. The scheme was developed by staff and students within their Equality, Diversity, and Inclusion Steering Group. The mentor scheme has been running for a year at the time of writing, and has been growing steadily. At first, mentor–mentee pairs were suggested to meet for up to six sessions, but feedback showed that between one and three online meetings were sufficient.

The content of the meetings between the mentor–student pairs included discussing identity, sharing experiences, strategies, and support, navigating practical issues, and signposting to organisations (e.g. the SLT Pride network). Students' feedback showed that the mentoring experience was positive: providing an opportunity to meet someone "like them", for example, with a similar background and experiences. The opportunity served to improve representation, to provide a role model who is pursuing the same career, and to learn about support networks. In fact, a range of issues were covered in meetings that were informal, friendly, unstructured, and relaxed.

Mentors fed back that they have enjoyed sharing their experiences and hearing about the latest equality and diversity opportunities for current students. Mentors and mentees have also provided constructive feedback that will help them to develop this scheme further.

The Leeds Beckett University team also invite their mentors to take part in equality, diversity, and inclusion events at the university, and to review aspects of their curriculum such as case studies. Mentors have also provided support to the university – for example, reviewing the admissions process (source: correspondence with Thiel, 2023).

Preceptorship

The period in which a speech and language therapy graduate transitions from student to autonomous practitioner is one area where there is a greater focus of research. In the US, this period is referred to as "clinical fellowship", and in the UK the term "preceptorship" has increasingly been adopted.

Darlene Robke (2016) describes the US clinical fellowship period in which speech and language pathologists are required to undertake a period of supervision and mentorship to support this transition. This article summarises Hudson's model (2010), which highlights the importance of the collaborative and reflective elements of this foundational stage in professional development, alongside observed practice and evaluation. In the UK, these elements may be expected of the preceptor role, where it exists. However, the mandated nature of the supervision and mentoring period in the US creates a tension with the voluntary nature of mentoring that is promoted in this book.

In a UK paper, Anderson (2001) proposed support and education in the transition period to "autonomous practitioner". At that point in time, the RCSLT recommended a mentor (not a line manager) to provide experienced support for the newly qualified SLT. Like the supervisor/mentor in today's US context, this role is fulfilled by the preceptor – assisting the newly qualified practitioner (NQP) with integrating theory and practice, building confidence, applying critical appraisal skills, and facilitating reflective practice, and helping the novice SLT to generate their own development goals. Anderson recommended that the mentor should receive additional training to build upon their existing practice educator skill set.

A further helpful perspective on the needs of the "novice" practitioner (after Dreyfus, 1986) is drawn from the US physical therapy (physiotherapy) profession. This paper identified the "desired components of a formal mentoring scheme for novice physical therapists" working in the outpatient therapy setting. The authors of the paper contrast the needs of the organisation with the needs of the mentee, and conclude that the latter should be the priority. Novice physical therapists themselves identified qualities in their mentors (and mentors in their mentees) that will be referred to again in Chapters 3 and 4, along with the challenges of setting up an organisational mentoring scheme.

Mentoring throughout the Stages of Career Progression

On its website, the RCSLT advocates the application of mentoring, primarily to "help you reach your goals at any stage of your career, by supporting you to learn new skills, overcome challenges at work and develop your confidence". For personal testimonies, it's worth reading Conrad (2006) about the impact of her mentors throughout her career as a speech and language pathologist in the US, and likewise Battle (2007). Doubtless, too, conversation with any mature SLT will equally reveal the "wise owls" who provided honest, encouraging, and challenging insights at key points throughout their own careers.

There are examples in the published literature where mentoring for specific clinical specialisms is recommended as part of the core service or employment offer. For example, working with Deaf and Hard of Hearing children (DeMoss et al., 2012); in an HIV rehabilitation programme (Solomon et al., 2011); and caring for those with primary progressive aphasia (Volkmer et al., 2022). An innovative approach to pre-registration education matches people with aphasia to mentor speech and language therapy students (Purves BA et al., 2013). However, these examples use the term "mentoring" for valuable and innovative roles that depart a little from the original definition set out in Chapter 1.

Research

SLTs whose careers take them into research roles were found to benefit from mentoring, which, according to Burger (2009), had been the "backbone" of the ASHA's Gathering Place initiative since 2004. The Mentoring Academic Research Careers (MARC) programme linked PhD students with researchers. It is common for researchers to be mentored by a peer who has a little more experience, or whose research is more advanced. It is even expected that mentoring is a core element of the role of a researcher. One speech and language therapy researcher that I heard from told me:

I have found it difficult to find someone who has the time to mentor me who is not personally invested i.e., supervisor/part of the research team. I think it's important to have separate mentors who you are not working directly with.

The Royal College of Speech and Language Therapists offers a matching scheme whereby SLTs working as clinical academics can access mentoring from another member. The network is:

> *designed to support speech and language therapists at all stages of a clinical academic career: from those who are just starting to consider carrying out practice-based projects or research, to those wishing to do a formal clinical-academic fellowship, and beyond.*
>
> (RCSLT website)

Leadership Development

Parsloe and Leedham (2000) promote transitional coaching for those who are moving into their first or subsequent leadership positions. They recommend that coach-mentors should have experience of holding leadership positions. This recommendation points to a mentor, rather than a pure coach, using the working definition of mentoring laid out in Chapter 1.

The RCSLT has a leadership mentor scheme whereby experienced leaders within the profession are appointed to support and guide other members of the profession, specifically to "'support with change and service transformation". As SLTs take up more senior or more formal leadership positions, it becomes more likely that they will consider approaching or identifying a mentor, perhaps seeking this sort of support for the first time since their student or newly qualified period. Beyond this profession, the value of mentors for leaders and aspiring senior leaders is very well recognised. The regional NHS Leadership Academies provide details of mentors (and coaches) who are available to provide support to other NHS employees on a pro bono (no-fee) basis.

In today's workplace, the emphasis on leadership being related to a position (for example a management role) has shifted in favour of leadership being an attribute. The regulator, the Health and Care Professions Council, now explicitly requires all registrants to understand leadership (Standard 8.6), recognise leadership skills

(Standard 8.7), identify "their own leadership qualities, behaviours and approaches, taking into account the importance of equality, diversity and inclusion" (Standard 8.7), and vitally, "demonstrate leadership behaviour appropriate to their practice" (HCPC, 2023). These standards apply to all SLTs regardless of the stage of their career or their position within an organisation or within the profession. Leadership is at the core of professionalism, therefore. Furthermore, leadership is a required component of the pre-registration curriculum delivered by universities.

In contrast, the term "executive coaching" has continued to be a primary offer of many professional coaching services. This offer of the coaching discipline suggests that the skills required of a practitioner who coaches the most senior leaders, form a different skill set from those who coach at undergraduate level (i.e., practice educators). And yet the skillset of the coach includes listening and asking carefully crafted questions. It is not clear whether executive leaders require a more sophisticated skillset, or mentors with executive leadership skills themselves, or whether it is the relative ability of senior leaders to pay for coaching that has resulted in this discipline emerging beyond the availability of mentoring for novice clinical practitioners.

I would suggest that, in order to fulfil the role of leader to the extent that our registration requires, SLTs at every level need to access the support, guidance, and encouragement of a mentor.

Resilience and Wellbeing

Older texts on coaching and mentoring rarely mention either resilience or wellbeing. In my own practice, conversations about resilience and emotional wellbeing increased significantly during the COVID-19 pandemic, when people's resilience was tested to extreme levels, and none more so than those in key worker roles like health and social care. The pressure on the speech and language therapy profession continued beyond the pandemic period, due to backlogs in service provision, increasing demand, expanding scope of speech and language therapy practice, and reduced staffing levels. The overall picture is one of a "'perfect storm" for the profession. It would not be at all appropriate for a mentor to focus on career development, learning, or transitioning into a new role without also considering the person's current and future wellbeing. My own understanding of resilience is not the ability to be unaffected by the blows that life throws at us, but instead the ability to bounce back. Or if not so much bouncing, at least recovering over time!

We cannot function optimally when we are in anything less than a state of wellbeing, and anything that detracts from that state will slow or halt progress towards our individual goals. Equally, recognising a state of "ill-being" may well be the trigger for an individual to seek mentoring support, or act as a catalyst for them seeking a career move or new opportunity.

As well as offering support in terms of resilience goals, an effective (and compassionate) mentor will ask the mentee to give feedback on their wellbeing at the outset and throughout the mentoring relationship, and agree goals that are informed by their wellbeing needs. For example, an adverse event that has rocked the person's wellbeing may be the reason for seeking their mentor's support or a new opportunity (e.g., a new job or retirement or a course of study). A mentor may flag the potential impact of a change of direction on the mentee's wellbeing. The mentor may encourage the mentee to consider how they can strengthen their resilience in readiness for a future planned transition. Finally, the maintenance of the mentoring relationship may be a key part of an individual's resilience plan.

Career Progression (and Workforce Recruitment and Retention)

At the time of writing, almost a quarter of SLT posts in the UK profession are vacant (RCSLT, 2023). A similar challenge faces the profession in the US, and Farquharson et al. (2022) describe the relationship between job dissatisfaction and vacancies and consequent wider workforce shortages, and advocate for "multi-tiered systems of support" in US public school SLP services. Mills (2008) noted that a "positive mentoring experience" was essential for a successful supervisory relationship. As a volunteer mentor with the Midlands NHS Leadership Academy, I have found that the most common reasons why healthcare colleagues reach out to seek a mentor are for support with reaching career goals, or because they find themselves at a career crossroads. The point at which it becomes clear that a change of direction, or at least a change of role, is the next step often triggers the question "Who can I turn to?", and at this point an independent guide who can provide a challenging and supportive coaching conversation is an obvious resource. Perhaps less commonly, we seek a mentor when we are new in a role. This is the point when a carefully selected person with relevant experience of the new territory that an SLT finds themselves in can really provide valuable advice and help us find our feet. While writing this book, I realised I had been in a new role for over six months, and it had not occurred to me before that I hadn't identified a new mentor myself! While some organisations will identify a buddy or a mentor to guide you through your early months in a new role, the benefits of identifying your own mentor beyond the induction or probation period will be covered in Chapter 3.

Pre-retirement

Whether an SLT ends their career because of long-term, thoughtful career and financial planning or in response to a personal change, which could be a change in the family situation such as caring for a relative or facing a deterioration in health, planning for retirement is preferable. However, in response to the workforce challenges described earlier in the chapter, the stresses that these place on experienced SLTs struggling to remain in post, and the challenges of adjusting to new demands, it is common for our most experienced colleagues to take retirement earlier than planned. The decision to end one's career, and to end it well, deserves equal consideration to any other career step. At this point, a person might consult someone with experience of completing their own career, or of taking steps towards retirement. Pre-retirement programmes are often provided by employers, but there are also mentors who specialise in pre-retirement planning.

Mentoring as an end-of-career option for SLTs – called legacy mentoring – is an option both for retired SLTs as mentors and for those seeking late career guidance.

Other professions have identified roles for those who have retired or are planning to retire: Mokgolodi (2022) developed a role for retired educators in Botswana. In the NHS, "legacy mentors" in their late careers support those who are at the start of their careers. Approximately a third of the NHS workforce are in the final third of their career. However, this has not been promoted as an opportunity for SLTs. I reached out to my professional network on social media as I was writing this section, and was unable to find any examples where this has been developed and maintained by any services, suggesting that there may be an untapped seam of mentoring ready to be explored. A range of options could be available to scale down a career and step back incrementally from paid employment. What a loss for our profession when those with more than 30 years of experience end their careers abruptly and with no consideration of how their knowledge and expertise could be shared with those at earlier career stages. This seems to me an ideal partnership between the newly retired and the newly qualified. There is great satisfaction in investing in the careers of a new generation of SLTs and leaving a legacy at the end of a long career. The newly retired or the soon-to-retire SLT is perhaps ideally equipped to provide that independent, expert guidance to a less experienced colleague that so many are seeking.

In Conclusion

Rolfe (2020) writes that "mentoring aims to facilitate self-development". As a facilitation of the mentee's learning, a mentor has a key role to play at any point in the SLT's career of continual development. Where there is learning, a mentor will have a role to enhance that learning. Operating in contexts that are in constant social, organisational, environmental, and technological change (termed VUCA – volatile, uncertain, complex, and ambiguous – by the US Army Heritage and Education Center, 2019), it is hard to conceive of a time in our careers when we are not required to continually adjust to new demands and drivers. The years immediately preceding the writing of this book have required us to adjust our practices in line with new insights about climate change, artificial intelligence, pandemic health risk, and inequities, by no means least in relation to race and ethnicity.

Learning is a lifelong journey, and a mentor – or a set of mentors – will support us to learn effectively from the challenges and experiences at every step of our SLT careers.

🔲 Ana's Story (Part 2)

Ana has spent several months accessing support to enable her to move forward after a difficult incident at work, which had left her emotionally bruised and lacking confidence in her own proven abilities. She had experienced some difficult feelings that echoed insecurities from her earlier life, which magnified the impact of the event itself. Some relationships in the workplace continue to be uncomfortable, although she has used reflective practice to move beyond them. Clinical supervision and counselling have both proven to be beneficial to her – in breaking the link between her negative self-beliefs and the proven achievements of her career up to the event and since it happened. The SLT Professional Lead in her organisation provided Ana with some valuable guidance and helped Ana to identify what her strengths are, reinforcing what Ana knows to be true, with objective evidence of what the Professional Lead has observed since Ana joined the service. Ana has now concluded that she wants to continue her career within the speech and language therapy profession. She believes it is now a good time to seek a change in direction – to identify what will be her next "chapter". She composes the following questions:

> "What opportunities or choices are available to me, to enable me to move into a different area of speech and language therapy?"
> "How can I play to my strengths as an SLT?"

Ana decides that she will find her own answers if another SLT who has suitable mentoring skills and a broad perspective of the profession can provide the space and time to coach her through these questions. An objective view would also be preferable, she concludes.

Considering the various people that Ana knows, she weighs up the options:

- an SLT in a leadership position in a larger department in a different, but nearby, organisation
- a tutor at the university where she studied
- the AHP lead in another county who happens to also be an SLT
- someone new – approach the professional body for guidance on a suggested person

Ana drafts a message that she can use to approach each of these colleagues:

Dear _____

I am a Band 5 speech and language therapist with three years' experience in acute inpatient settings, and I now find myself at a career crossroads. Having explored my position thoughtfully, I remain committed to a career in speech and language therapy, but would like to identify my next steps and options.

I feel your overview of the profession and the wider context would really help me take my decision. I do appreciate that other commitments may make this difficult. While I realise you must be extremely busy, I wonder if you would be able to offer me a mentoring conversation to help me reach a decision?

Best wishes

Ana

🔔 Recap

A mentor could add value at any stage of your career, and especially at career transition points such as:

- selecting a career in speech and language therapy
- deciding where to apply to study
- resilience through the pre-registration period – as a student
- on placement in a specific clinical setting
- preparing to apply for first position as a registered SLT
- settling into the first position after registration
- preparing to make the transition into a new role or specialism
- considering promotion or a change in direction
- undertaking a new venture, such as research or further education
- providing support through a difficult period – where health, well-being, workload, work relationships, or personal situations challenge us to keep going
- preparation for retirement or a complete change of career

💭 Reflection Prompts

You may find it helpful to pause now to reflect on and note:

- Who provided me with the advice and information I needed when I first took the decision to apply for a place at University to study speech and language therapy?
- What attributes in a mentor do I consider most important to support my career development at that point?
- Since then, who else has encouraged me, challenged me, recognised my strengths, and believed in me? To whom have I turned at points when I needed some additional wisdom and guidance?

- Note the names of your mentors at different stages of your career.

- Who else do you consider may be willing to be approached now, and when you next need that input?

- Do I have an opportunity to support others within my profession, and what might be the longer-term benefit of doing so? How might this support their development? How might this support my development? How might this benefit the wider profession and the people who will access our services?

- Given a lack of evidence in this area, are there ways in which I could develop or evaluate mentoring in my setting?

- In Matthews et al. (2021), university study students were randomly allocated to a peer mentor. How important is self-selection in the mentoring relationship? How feasible is it to support self-selection for a whole cohort of students? How might I match mentors with mentees in my service/course/team?

Action Plan

Enquirers	Mentors
Early Career	
Who is encouraging me and answering my questions about a future career and about my options for studying?	Do I have the skills to support decision making in an enquirer?
	How could I develop those skills?
Does my university provide a mentoring scheme?	How might I contribute to the wider profession?
Does my employer provide a mentoring scheme?	How might I support an enquirer's career choices?
	What are my development opportunities?
	Do I know where to find information or resources outside my own experiences?

Next steps

What …

How …

When …

What do I hope to learn from the remaining chapters of this book?

Mid-career	
Who are the key people who have invested in my career development so far?	Do I have the skills to support decision making in an enquirer?
	How could I develop those skills?
Who do I turn to when I need a listening ear or some advice?	How might I contribute to the wider profession?
What is the next career decision or dilemma that I can see approaching?	How might I support an enquirer's career choices?
What conversation do I want to have at my next appraisal/review? How can I prepare to get the impact I'm looking for?	What are my development opportunities?
	Do I know where to find information or resources outside my own experiences?

Next steps

What …

How …

When …

What do I hope to learn from the remaining chapters of this book?

Late Career	
How well developed are my retirement plans? Who can support me with creating a plan or preparing for retirement? What legacy would I want to leave behind me before I end my career? How could I plan to achieve that legacy? Who can I approach to discuss this?	What opportunities do I have to support the development of younger colleagues before or after I retire? Who might I approach to offer my services? What training would I need? Where could I source that?
Next steps What … How … When … What do I hope to learn from the remaining chapters of this book?	
Try working through the questions for mentors now – maybe you have something to offer others.	Try working through the questions for enquirers now – maybe you have something to gain from others.

 Further Reading

American Speech and Hearing Association (ASHA) website: https://www.asha.org/students/mentoring/

 References

Anderson, H. (2001) Clinical teaching and mentoring: Vital in the development of competent therapists. *International Journal of Language and Communication Disorders*, 36, 138.

American Speech and Hearing Association. ASHA's mentoring programs. Available from: https://www.asha.org/students/mentoring/ [accessed on 27/10/2023].

Atherton, M., Davidson, B. and McAllister, L. (2017) Exploring the emerging profession of speech-language pathology in Vietnam through pioneering eyes. *International Journal of Speech-Language Pathology*, 19 (2), 109–120.

Battle, D. (2007) Mentoring: The cycle of caring. *ASHA Leader*, 12 (2), 12.

Benner, P. (1982) From novice to expert. *American Journal of Nursing*, 82 (3), 402–407.

Brown, L. (2023) Personal communication [email] Sent to M. *Heritage*, 19 October.

Buning, M. and Buning, S. (2019) *Beyond Supervised Learning: A Multi-perspective Approach to Outpatient Physical Therapy Mentoring*. Augusta, GA: Taylor and Francis.

Burger, S. (2009) *'Gathering Place' Celebrates Five Years of Service: Mentoring Programs Link Clinicians, Students, Faculty, and Researchers*. Rockville, MD: American Speech-Language-Hearing Association.

Conrad, B. (2006) An SLP reaches out to mentors, gives back to students. *ASHA Leader*, 11 (13), 57–58.

DeMoss, W. L., Clem, B. C. and Wilson, K. (2012) Using technology to mentor aspiring LSLS professionals. *Volta Review*, 112 (3), 329–343.

Dreyfus, H. L. and Dreyfus, S. E. (1986) *Mind over Machine: The Power of Human Intuition and Expertise in the Age of the Computer*. Oxford: Basil Blackwell.

Farquharson, K., Therrien, M., Barton-Hulsey, A. and Brandt, A. F. (2022) How to recruit, support, and retain speech-language pathologists in public schools. *Journal of School Leadership*, 32 (3), 225–245.

Greene, S. M. (2021) Effects of a peer-mentoring program on speech-language pathology graduate student stress. *Perspectives of the ASHA Special Interest Groups*, 6 (4), 855–866.

HCPC. (2023) https://www.hcpc-uk.org/globalassets/resources/standards/standards-of-proficiency---speech-and-language-therapists.pdf

Health Education England's RePAIR. (2018) https://www.hee.nhs.uk/news-blogs-events/news/health-education-england-gains-valuable-insight-improving-student-retention

Hudson, M (2010) Supervision to mentoring: Practical considerations. *Perspectives on Administration and Supervision*, 20 (2), 71–75.

Kent, J. and McDonald, S. (2021) What are the experiences of Speech and Language therapists implementing a staff development approach in early years settings to enhance good communication practices? *Child Language Teaching and Therapy*, 37 (1), 85–97.

Kent, R. D. (2006) The power of passionate mentoring: Mentoring: Person-to-person professional development. *The ASHA Leader*, 11 (12), 26.

Kline, N. (1998) *Time to Think: Listening to Ignite the Human Mind*. London: Cassell.

Lewis, K. S. (2015) Stepping out of your zone. *ASHA Leader*, 20 (2), 42–46.

Mak, S., Hunt, M., Boruff, J., Zaccagnini, M. and Thomas, A. (2022) Exploring professional identity in rehabilitation professions: A scoping review. *Advances in Health Sciences Education: Theory and Practice*, 27 (3) 1–23.

Matthews, J., Perryman, T. and Kneiss, D. (2021) Undergraduate student success initiatives in communication sciences and disorders. *Perspectives of the ASHA Special Interest Groups*, 6 (3), 601–609.

McPherson, K., Kersten, P., George, S., Lattimer, V., Breton, A., Ellis, B., Kaur, D. and Frampton, G. (2006) A systematic review of evidence about extended roles for allied health professionals. *Journal of Health Services Research and Policy*, 11 (4), 240–247.

Mills, C. (2007) *Career Coach: How to Plan Your Career and Land Your Perfect Job UK*. Bath: Trotman.

Mills, K. (2008) Benefits and characteristics of mentoring students and young professionals. *Perspectives on Administration and Supervision*, 18 (2), 67–73.

Mokgolodi, H. L. (2022) Retired educators' career transitin as a new life role of underwriting career development in Botswana. *Journal of Population Ageing*, 15 (4), 891–905.

Naidoo, K., Yuhaniak, H., Borkoski, C., Levangie, P. and Abel, Y. (2021) Networked mentoring to promote social belonging among minority physical therapist students and develop faculty cross-cultural psychological capital. *Mentoring and Tutoring: Partnership in Learning*, 29 (5), 586–606.

Parsloe, E. and Leedham, M. (2000) *Coaching and Mentoring: Practical Techniques for Developing Learning and Performance*. London: Kagan

Purves, B. A., Petersen, J. and Purveen, G. (2013) An aphasia mentoring program: Perspectives of speech-language pathology students and of mentors with aphasia. *American Journal of Speech-Language Pathology*, 22 (2), S370–S379.

Quigley, D., Loftus, L., McGuire, A. and O'Grady, K. (2020) An optimal environment for placement learning: Listening to the voices of speech and language therapy students. *International Journal of Communication Disorders*, 55 (4), 506–519.

RCSLT Clinical Academic Mentors Resource. Available from: https://www.rcslt.org/search/?search-query=clinical+academic+mentors&page= [accessed on 3/10/2023].

Robke, D. D. (2016) Foundational resources and terminology for supervision and mentorship. *Perspectives of the ASHA Special Interest Groups*, 11 (2), 1. American Speech and Hearing Association.

Rodriguez, J. C. (2016) Our clients are diverse: Why aren't we? *ASHA Leader*, 21 (5), 40–42.

Rolfe, A. (2020) *Mentoring Mindset, Skills, and Tools* (4th edition). SouthWest Rocks, NSW: Mentoring Works.

Royal College of Speech and Language Therapists (2023) Vacancy rates reach 23% in Speech and language therapy. Available from: https://www.rcslt.org/news/vacancy-rates-reach-23-in-speech-and-language -therapy/ [accessed on 18/6/2023].

Saenz, T. I. (2000) Issues in recruitment and retention of graduate students. *Communication Disorders Quarterly*, 21 (4), 246–250.

Solomon, P., O'Brien, K., Hard, J., Worthington, C., Zack, E. and Gopee, N. (2011) An HIV mentorship programme for rehabilitation professionals: Lessons learned from a pilot initiative. *International Journal of Therapy and Rehabilitation*, 18 (5), 280–289.

Theil, L. (2023) Mentor scheme information [email] Sent to M. Heritage, 28 June.

Tucker, J. (2013) When to bring in your supervisor. *The ASHA Leader* 18 (12), 28–29.

US Army Heritage & Education Center (2019) Available from: Who first originated the term VUCA (Volatility, Uncertainty, Complexity and Ambiguity)? - USAHEC Ask Us a Question (libanswers.com) [accessed on 16/5/2023].

Volkmer, A., Cartwright, J., Ruggero, L., Beales, A., Gallée, J., Grasso, S., Henry, M., Jokel, R., Kindell, J., Khayum, R., Pozzebon, M., Rochon, E., Taylor-Rubin, C., Townsend, R., Walker, F., Beeke, S. and Hersh, D. (2022) Principles and philosophies for speech and language therapists working with people with primary progressive aphasia: An international expert consensus. *Disability and Rehabilitation*, 45 (6), 1–16.

Wright-Harp, W. and Cole, P. A. (2008) A mentoring model for enhancing success in graduate education. *Contemporary Issues in Communication Science and Disorders*, 35 (Spring), 4–16.

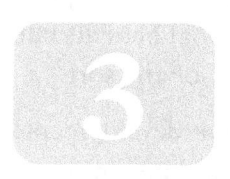

How to Find and Work with Your Mentor

Introduction

This chapter will cover:

1. how to secure a mentor by:

    - identifying potentially suitable people to mentor you

    - deciding on the best way to make an effective initial approach – a positive opening conversation

    - deciding whether the relationship is likely to be beneficial to you

2. how to get the best results from the mentoring relationship

How to Secure a Mentor

As we are seeing in Ana's story, she considered potential mentors she already knew and might have an insight into her own situation.

A mentor needs:

- **Capacity** – the time to devote to you and your development. While this may not be a large commitment, if they cannot find time to prioritise meeting with you, you will not benefit from what they have to offer.

DOI: 10.4324/9781003386827-4

- **Altruism** – an interest in developing others, without an immediate reward. Motivation is distinct from reward. In my own experience, all my mentors gained some reciprocal personal benefit, but I did not pay any of them or agree to an exchange of any sort.

- **Motivation** to invest in *you* and to support *your* development. Maybe there is an existing relationship, or else they have an interest in a community of which you are a representative. Or maybe your approach will appeal to something from their own story. It may also be that the mentor has a need of their own that they believe you will be able to support them with. For example, they may want to understand more of your situation to help them in their own development. You may never discover all of the motivations of your mentor, but it's important to realise that your mentor will be considering these.

- **Listening skills** – good leaders should already have these, but may not! Anyone who promotes themselves as a coach should be able to use active listening as a way of developing another person. Nowadays, it is more common to expect some listening/coaching skills in leaders.

- **Resources** – the ideal mentor, in addition to the above attributes, will have something to signpost you toward. This might be introductions to people in their network who can help you in different ways, or recommending reading or courses to help you develop yourself. At the point of approaching them, you may not know what resources they have to offer – most experienced leaders have a lot more than meets the eye! It would be wise to select your mentor primarily for their altruistic interest in you and their good coaching skills rather than for the resources they can provide you with.

Here are some examples from my own mentoring experiences:

One very senior manager who had insight into the ways our organisation operated was able to help me negotiate barriers that I'd encountered. Most of these didn't seem as ominous from the mentor's perspective as they appeared to me. I believe that their mentoring of me may also have helped them understand how the organisation was experienced by its employees.

An external mentor was interested in developing connections in the sector in which I worked to enable them to fulfil a vacancy in their own board.

A peer from another region was asked to sit on the interview panel for a promotion I secured, and afterwards asked to be introduced to me. We later mentored one another ("reciprocal mentoring" – more in Chapter 5) at different stages in our respective careers. Initially, I benefited from their experience and interest in me as I settled into my new role. Later we embarked, at different times, on the same development programme, and we mentored one another through this period of study.

It is perhaps the best starting point to ascertain whether someone has the capacity (within their working week) and subsequently confirm their altruism, motivation, skills, and resources.

I mentor people who work in the NHS in my region. Partly this is to help me stay in touch with the healthcare sector now that I am one step removed, working in a university. But mainly, there is a genuine motivation to "put something back" now that I have moved on in my own career, but I take a wealth of experience with me, combined with a more objective perspective.

Identifying Potentially Suitable People to Mentor You

Figure 3.1 shows how wide the scope of your mentoring search could be. Digital technology enables us to connect easily across the world – with time zones being more of a barrier than geographical distance. In relation to six mentors: One was part of my current network. One worked within a wider local health system, but had moved beyond my network. Two were from the wider allied health professional (AHP)/ healthcare network. Two others were not part of even a wider professional or personal network. Mapping my own six mentors against the four zones in Figure 3.1 shows that the mentors that have had the most influence in my own career came from beyond my own current network (the people I know and encounter on a regular basis). Clearly,

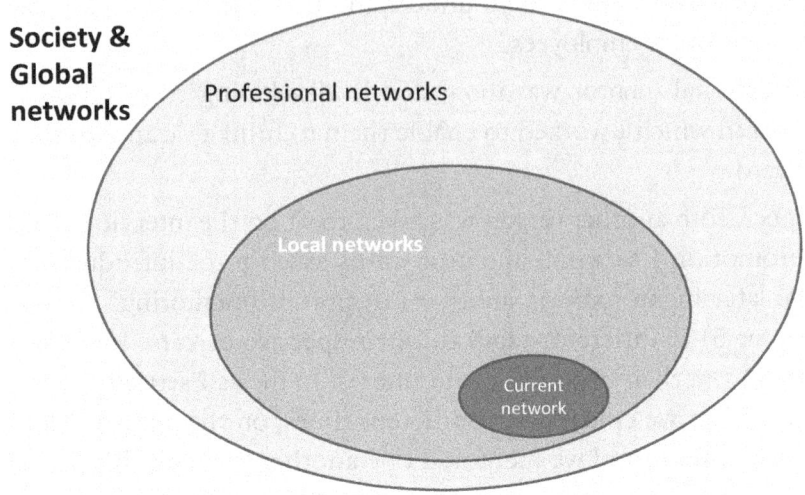

Figure 3.1 Finding a mentor through your networks

finding the right mentor requires casting the net wider than day-to-day contacts.

Current network – your first step will probably be to consider who you know already. The benefit of approaching someone who is already in your day-to-day work environment is that they are accessible, know you well, and importantly, understand the context in which you currently work. One of my own mentors, T, helped me understand the internal political context I was working within. T also suggested that B might support me with my new role. However, the potential drawback of only searching among the people you already know is a lack of objectivity and broader perspective.

Scoping the **wider local networks** takes a little more effort, but may provide you with the fresh eyes that you need:

• **Health and social care and local authorities** – integrated care systems form collaborations across the sectors and provide opportunities for you to make connections with local leaders outside your organisation. This could help to understand the local system and its opportunities better.

- **Universities** – tutors and academics in your local universities are connected to wider professional networks through research and practice education and may offer a useful step away from your own situation.

- **Allied health professions** – these are now organised into AHP councils and faculties. By finding out who represents the AHPs in your system, you may be able to access an AHP mentor locally, and beyond the sector you work within.

- **Wider speech and language therapy networks (e.g., non-statutory sector providers)** – there are likely to be multiple providers of speech and language therapy services in the local area – those who work with a different client group or clinical field may offer new insight and have different networks within the local profession. These may include not-for-profit organisations, sole trader businesses, and growing independent practices.

Professional networks may include:

- **Professional bodies** – the Royal College of Speech and Language Therapists (RCSLT) provides a powerful network across the speech and language therapy profession, with very high proportions of registered speech and language therapists (SLTs) in the UK maintaining their membership. Access to specific networks through clinical excellence networks and regional hubs and through leadership mentors could help to find a person within the profession with the experience you are seeking.

- **Clinical specialisms** – there is evidence of mentoring by clinical specialists being effective. Examples include:
  - physiotherapy – see Buning and Buning (2019)
  - SLTs working with people with primary progressive aphasia – see Volkmer et al. (2022)
  - community SLTs practising in adult dysphagia in South Africa – see Coutts (2019)

- **AHP forum** – there are online platforms that support professional networking around specific interest areas across the allied health professions. These provide useful ways to build communities of practice around clinical and professional interest areas.

- **NHS coaching and mentoring database** – nowadays, the people I mentor tend to find me on a regional database coordinated by the NHS Leadership Academy in my region. This provides an opportunity for an SLT to browse through the profiles of available mentors seeking a match for the profession, clinical interests, organisational position, or experience they are looking for. The approach is made via the platform and appears as a notification in the mentor's email inbox. There remains the opportunity to add a personal introduction, like Ana's. This facility is available in many NHS regions, and is a helpful way to find someone who has an interest in and experience of mentoring.

Society/Global Networks

With digital technology, our networking is not limited by the need to travel. Reciprocal relationships between professionals whose experience crosses traditional boundaries – nationality, profession, or seniority – offer great potential benefits. We will explore this further in Chapter 5. I was interested to reflect on the professional backgrounds of the six people I have identified as my mentors: business, NHS management, nursing, and three allied health professionals (two physiotherapists, an ophthalmologist, and just one SLT).

Why would we limit our search for a mentor to our local area, our own profession, or the sector we currently work in? I hope that over time our profession will extend its networking beyond the UK so that we can learn from, and support, one another within the global profession. We will explore this a little further in Chapter 5.

DeMoss et al. (2012) write about the global shortage of professionals who support children who are Deaf and Hard of Hearing and their families "who are seeking listening and spoken language" outcomes. Their global initiative provided mentoring to retain and develop professions within this niche.

In Chapter 6, I will return to a vision for a future where perhaps culture, nationality, and geography are no longer barriers to impactful mentoring relationships.

In Chapters 1 and 2, we started to hear Ana's story. In this account, Ana considered:

- who understands the wider scope of her individual professional situation – in her case, this was the world of speech and language therapy

- who is outside her immediate organisation – to ensure objectivity and confidentiality

- who has no conflicts of interest in her next career move – independence from her situation

She then considered the wider profession in the region beyond the system in which she works. Our profession is a small one, and being confident that a mentor is independent and objective, as well as well-informed, is a challenge. Ana identified that she wanted to find someone within the profession but outside her current network. She is not limited to the speech and language therapy profession in her own region, but she believes that she will get the most out of an initial meeting if it is face-to-face, and therefore travelling distance restricts her.

Ana arrived at the qualities/attributes to complete a "Mentor Spec". For her current purposes, the clinical or non-clinical specialism or the setting in which they work is less important. Ana is looking outside the speech and language therapy profession, for the following:

- suitable mentoring skill

- a broad perspective of the profession

- the space and time to work through her questions (or "dilemmas")

- an objective view, therefore outside her own sphere

She doesn't therefore limit her search to those with experience of her clinical specialism (adults with acquired conditions) or the setting she works in (acute inpatients).

Ana considered approaching the RCSLT for signposting to other potential mentors beyond her current knowledge. Although she has not yet met two of the people on her shortlist (SLTs in leadership positions outside her organisation), she might have gone further in her research – for example, asking colleagues to suggest people in their networks. However, her need for privacy about her current career crossroads made her reluctant to share this.

She identifies three people to approach from beyond her current network:

- **her wider local speech and language therapy network** – a tutor at the university where she studied and an SLT in a leadership position

- **the wider professional network** – the AHP lead in another county

Ana also considers a fourth option: to approach the professional body for guidance on a suggested person.

She writes to Kim, the AHP lead in another county who happens to also be an SLT.

A Positive Opening Conversation

In her first approach, Ana provides each potential mentor with sufficient information to help them decide whether they are willing to meet her. Her approach is brief (people are busy, and may not read the whole of a long introduction) and she makes it by email. It is also personal; she uses their name. She also includes some key information:

- her profession and career stage

- her dilemma and her question

- her "ask" – an initial meeting with an explicit aim (accessing mentoring)

From this email, the recipient would completely understand what Ana wants, without her having to describe the intricacies of her recent experiences and her future options. The lack of detail may even intrigue them.

Ana's approach allows the recipient to:

- take time to consider and respond (unlike a phone call)
- decide whether they feel drawn to help her and whether they have capacity (time) and capability (resources and skills) to meet her needs

It would be much easier to decline her invitation at this point than after an initial meeting, and after she has disclosed her situation.

I recommend being open and using the term "mentoring". To be asked to be a mentor indicates a level of respect for the person's experience. The word implies an opportunity to help someone move forward in their life. There are some universal understandings of the essence of mentoring even though the detail of how a mentoring relationship may play out in practice will need further discussion.

Finally, Ana's tone is respectful – and hopeful.

An Introductory Conversation

This may be called a "chemistry meeting", "pre-conversation", or "first meeting" – because it could be thought of as an opportunity to see whether there is a reciprocal positive feeling about a future mentoring relationship. The first conversation is as likely to be on the phone or online as it is to be face-to-face.

Whatever we call it, the first conversation is an opportunity for both parties to make an early decision about whether they feel sufficiently positive about the aims and form of a mentoring relationship. In pressurised professional life, neither mentor nor mentee will have the time to spend on an unfruitful relationship, so it is vital to have a frank discussion about whether it is likely to be what both want to invest in.

What to expect:

Informality – both the mentor and the person seeking mentoring (mentee) need to get to know one another and to see how the conversation feels. Mentoring requires trust, and both parties are finding out whether they could trust the other. As a mentee, you will be exposing some vulnerabilities to the mentor, and it is important to sense that you will not be judged nor misunderstood. The mentor's listening behaviour in this first meeting will be very important to establish the trust needed. This goes beyond a guarantee of confidentiality. Carl Rogers' concept of "unconditional positive regard" (Rogers, 1951) as the basis of a person-centred therapeutic interaction is relevant here. Peltier (2010, 105) helpfully describes it: "'I'll accept you as you are' rather than 'I'll accept you when'".

This subjective sense of the mentor making the mentee feel sufficiently comfortable to disclose insecurities and vulnerabilities is an indicator of their trustworthiness. This could only be ascertained through informal conversation, in which both parties share a little of their background and the reasons behind their interests in the relationship.

This first encounter may feel more of an exploratory chat than a formal process. However, be prepared to be asked questions that may feel challenging. A good coach asks carefully crafted questions as well as listening attentively. If the mentor asks you a question that makes you think (and gives you a new insight into your situation), this too is an indication of their skill.

An overview of the situation or circumstances – each of you will benefit from gaining an understanding of the other's current and previous roles and any other mentoring experience. Be prepared to share something of your personal circumstances. This is not as inappropriate as you might initially think. The mentor is looking at you as a whole person, not just what happens at work. So many of our drivers, detractors, blind spots, and aspirations relate to factors beyond our employment or occupation. Be ready to share more about yourself if you are asked. The mentor may share less of themselves. That is appropriate. It would be easy to lapse into a cosy chat. The focus is on what the mentee needs.

Motivation – The mentor will be offering their services for altruistic reasons. But as a mentee, you will be interested to listen out and understand what is motivating your mentor. Is there something about the mentee that connects with the mentor's values or background, for example? Or maybe the mentor might be hoping to gain more insight into the context in which the mentee works. The focus of the initial conversation, however, will be the motivation of the mentee:

- the reason they are looking for mentoring
- their aspirations, goals, and objectives toward which mentoring may help
- their understanding of mentoring – what it is and is not (see Chapter 1)
- the reason they have approached this mentor in the first place – by recommendation or reputation – and is their expectation of the mentor's experience or influence realistic?

Decision – Be prepared to make the decision on the spot. This shouldn't be something that either party needs to think about at length. At least, if you need to think about it, you are probably going to decline pursuing the relationship further. If you don't feel comfortable to progress mentoring with this mentor, then feel confident to give a reason and not occupy any more of their time. For example:

> *Thank you for your time. This meeting has been so helpful. I now realise that I'd not completely understood your current role/I had been mistakenly thought you had a background in …/I've been looking for help with … but I now realise that this isn't your focus. Without wasting your time further, I'd just like to thank you again.*

As you have made the initial approach, it is appropriate that you will make the decision, and with confidence. If you don't feel comfortable, then the mentor probably won't either. A final point is that saving someone else time is never bad news for them!

In most situations, the decision is a positive one about future mentoring, especially if there has been an introductory email that the mentor has already considered. In these cases, one party may conclude the initial conversation along the lines of:

> *Well, having heard everything you've shared and what you're hoping to achieve in the future, I would like to offer you any help that I can. If you still think I can help you, I'd be happy to put another date in the diary.*

or

> *thank you so much for your time today. If you are still interested, I'd very much like to take you up on any offer of support that you are able to offer me. What are your thoughts?*

Practicalities – Blanchard and Diaz-Ortiz (2017) refer to the discussions covered above as the "essence" meeting – "A successful first meeting with a potential mentor or mentee puts the person before the tactical … or essence before form".

Assuming that the relationship is going ahead, the practical issues (i.e., the tactical) or "form" will need to be agreed at the end of the meeting. As a minimum, try to keep the momentum you've just built by pinning down the next meeting:

- will meetings be in-person or by video call (e.g., Teams, Zoom)? What will be the preferred place for in-person meetings (e.g. on work premises or in a neutral place such as a coffee shop)?
- what are the best times of day?
- what are the preferred days of the week?
- length of session – this might be at least an hour, depending on the mentor's preference.

- what preparation is expected of the mentee?

- will the mentor expect to agree a "contract" (see Chapter 4)?

- is there any other information that the mentee could helpfully share – e.g., would the mentor prefer to receive anything in advance of a meeting?

In respect of these considerations, the mentee should expect to do most of the work, including travel. The mentor may not be able to fit this role into their working day and so the mentee should also expect to be flexible with their own time – with the agreement of their employer if work time is likely to be used for mentoring meetings.

And finally, if the first meeting is particularly successful, the mentoring may even be well underway already!

Working with a Mentor

We have considered at length how to identify, approach, and meet your mentor. Before we cover how to be a great mentor, we will consider how to be mentored. My own experiences of being mentored, and of being a mentor, have brought the following six principles into focus in order for both mentor and mentee to get the most out of the precious time you are about to share.

Prepare

At your first conversation, you will have shared something of your "dilemma", the challenge or problem that led you to seek a mentor. Having identified your overarching problem, working with a mentor is one of your strategies. Each session should work tactically towards resolving that problem or dilemma. You should come to your planned meetings with a clear idea of what it is you want to achieve next. As a mentor, I ask for a "coaching question" near the start of each session. This often takes the form "How can I ...?", and examples are shown in Table 3.1.

Table 3.1 Examples of how to express a dilemma into a question to consider with a mentor

Dilemma	Strategy	Tactics – Example Questions (Session Aims)
I'm in the wrong job	Working with my mentor to move into a new field	"**How can I** work out what my next step will be?"
		"**How can I** decide which jobs to apply for?"
		"**How can I** maximise my chance of success at interview?"
I've just moved into a new role, and I want to make an impact	Working with my mentor to develop my leadership	"**How can I** understand more about the way the organisation works?"
		"**How can I** communicate with my team, more confidently?"
		"**How can I** learn more about leadership?"
I'm struggling with relationships at work	Working with my mentor to be more effective within the organisation	"**How can I** understand the power dynamics here?"
		"**How can I** maintain my resilience and wellbeing in the meantime?"
		"**How can I** have a positive impact on working relationships?"
I'm keen to develop specialist clinical skills in …	Working with my mentor to improve my clinical capabilities	"**How can I** find the up-to-date evidence base?"
		"**How can I** critically review my clinical practice in this field?"
		"**How can I** further enhance my knowledge and understanding of the field?"
I'm midway through my SLT training and wondering if I can succeed	Working with my mentor to maintain my motivation and stamina	"**How can I** be better organised to complete my assignments on time?"
		"**How can I** use reflective practice as a learning tool?"
		"**How can I** decide in which area of speech and language therapy I want to start my career?"

I like this form of question:

"How" – opens positive thinking (rather than "Can I?")

"can" – leads us into considering possibilities

"I" – focuses on the person who is responsible for achieving their overall goal

My practice has been greatly influenced by Claire Pedrick (2021), who uses the opening question 'What would you like to think about today?'

Your mentor may prefer you to send this question in advance. Coming prepared to open the session with a focus will help both of you use the time to best advantage. That means more time is devoted to thinking about the answer, and less about the question. There is a temptation to spend time recapping progress made since your previous meeting. However, a word of caution about this: mentoring meetings do not usually happen frequently, and so bringing your mentor up to date can use time that could be devoted instead to considering your new question. Consider whether a brief email (bullet points) could cover this outside the meeting. It's also worth deciding how much of the detail your mentor needs to know. They will be curious about the impact that the mentoring is having on your development, but the focus of each session should be forward thinking.

Engage

By "engage", I mean that you participate fully and actively in your own mentoring sessions. The mentor is engaged in mentoring you, but what is the verb for "being mentored" (a passive concept)? Maybe it is "thinking" (Pedrick, 2021), or maybe "learning". While the mentor will be listening and asking questions, and maybe remarking on what they notice about you as you talk, the bulk of the "work" will be yours. That may mean that you are doing most of the talking, but there may also be silences. In my experience, when the mentor asks a question and the mentee stops, looks away, and is quiet, this indicates that they are finding new insights. A good mentor will wait to hear what these are.

Engagement may also mean:

- making notes

- asking for information ("In your experience …?")

- asking for signposting ("What resources have you found useful?")

- asking for guidance ("What would you recommend?")

- asking for an introduction ("Do you know of anyone else I could approach?")

- summarising your next steps

Be Challenged

You have chosen your mentor to help you develop. Part of that will be to provide a safe space in which they challenge you. This may be by providing you with feedback:

- "When you said that, I noticed …"

- "I notice that your energy has dipped a little when we started to talk about that …"

Be prepared to consider what they observe and what it tells you.

Mentors also may start to challenge you more directly:

- "When we set out on this, you seemed ambitious to achieve the goal, I'm wondering if that is still the case?"

- "You said that your team don't back you – but I wonder what *your* responsibility is?"

- "You felt that the exam was unfair – but was there anything more that you could have done, maybe?"

- "So, what have you learned from all of that?"

Reflect

Reflective practice is a core part of our continuing professional development, and a range of reflective cycles are available to guide us, from describing an event through to planning how to improve our practice in future – examples include Kolb's (1984), Gibbs' (1988), and Driscoll's (2007) reflective cycles.

Reflection after the session is a vital part of the mentoring process. It's good practice to block out the time as soon as possible after your scheduled time with your mentor. This will give you the opportunity to consolidate your learning and your new insights and to commit to the actions you need to take.

You will probably also undertake reflection within the mentoring session. This may be in the "quiet" moments when new insights emerge – what Pedrick calls the "transformational shift" (2021). I recommend Nancy Kline's (1998) work again here: her proposal is that a facilitator can provide a learning environment in which a person can think, and this applies well to the mentoring session. Some prefer to reflect in silence with a pen and paper; others with a voice note, or while they are active (walking or exercising). Some like to talk and reflect, and these external processors may discover that significant insights occur during conversations with their mentor.

It could be helpful to share with your mentor where your breakthrough moments most often occur, and whether you are comfortable with silent reflection in the session or prefer to keep talking.

Good, or even essential, practice is to identify somewhere to record your mentoring – where to jot things down during the session and return to them later. It's helpful to make a structured reflective entry (using your preferred model) soon after the mentoring session. This will lead you into "next steps" or actions to review before you embark on the next session. Reading back over previous reflections can provide you with an overview of the progress you have made during the mentoring journey.

Follow Up

The next steps or actions are the outputs of reflection. Without the discipline of reflecting on what happened and what you learned during each mentoring meeting, you will not gain full benefit from the session. Further questions such as "So what?" help you to build on the learning that started to emerge, and "What next?" defines the output – consolidating the new learning into action. Making that shift into action demonstrates commitment that justifies your mentor's investment in you. The progress happens in between the sessions, and not within them. Your follow-up actions do not need to be world-changing. Examples are searching online for further resources, booking a place on a webinar or course, approaching someone for further information, or reading a book or article and reflecting on it – in other words, completing further self-directed continuing professional development activity.

Appreciate

Like any other relationship, this one will be expected to grow over time as you learn about one another, and as your level of trust builds. We each have our preferences for how appreciation is shown to us. By understanding the motivations of your mentor (see the section "An Introductory Conversation"), you may identify tangible ways to show that you value their support. For example, from my own experience: one mentor gained new insights into the organisation from mentoring a more junior colleague; another engaged in reciprocal mentoring with me over several years. If your mentor is explicit about their own motivations, you may be able to share something of value with them. Your mentor is investing in your development, and any feedback that shows how you can link a new insight, some progress in your situation, or a change in your thinking with their mentoring will provide them with encouragement and feedback. Almost too obvious to put into print: keep saying "Thank you" in any way you can. Mentors give their time, thought, and energy to you, altruistically, and your appreciation is important.

Ana's Story (Part 3)

Dear Kim,

Thank you so much for making time to meet with me yesterday. I found it really helpful when you prompted me to summarise my current dilemma in a succinct question. Your follow-up questions were incisive and insightful!

During the first session with you, I learned that I am feeling drawn toward a possible future research career. I've made a plan of my next steps, which I'd like to share with you here, to keep me accountable for moving forward:

- Approach the Research and Development lead in my Trust.
- Ask to shadow the Audit and Quality committee.
- Go and talk to the hospital librarians.
- Explore RCSLT and AHP researcher networks.
- Sign up for the regional research newsletter.
- Explore the option of a master's research degree and explore the funding options.

I've now found and completed the AHP career choice tool that you mentioned but couldn't locate. It's actually at https://ahpcareers .co.uk/ if you need it again. And I've also offered to write a short piece on Acute Speech and Language Therapy and dysphagia for our Integrated Care system careers website, which was lacking much coverage of our profession.

You very kindly offered to introduce me to a colleague in your department who leads on postgraduate research opportunities. We agreed that when I've completed all the above steps (or got stuck!), I will get back in touch to share my progress, and if it seems appropriate, I would really appreciate a follow-up meeting,

Until then, thank you so much 😊

Ana

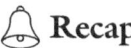 Recap

Sometimes, we approach someone and ask them to mentor us. More often, perhaps, we are drawn to individuals who invest time and interest in our development, and only later look back and view them as a "mentor". One of my mentors shared the term "Wise Owls" as the people we turn to in our careers when we are seeking direction or a new approach.

We can cast the net wide when we are seeking a mentor. Considering the experience and objectivity we want, there is a wealth of networks and platforms that we as AHPs and SLTs can access to find the right person.

A careful approach and introductory meeting will help both parties discern whether this is a relationship that could bear fruit – ideally reciprocally.

Making the most of mentoring involves: preparation, engagement, being challenged, reflection, and follow-up. Showing appreciation is good courtesy to your mentor.

💬 Reflection Prompts

You may find it helpful to pause now to reflect on and note:

- During your own career, who can you identify as the "Wise Owls" whose guidance and time resulted in you taking successful steps forward?

- What do you reflect was important about their approach? Their experience? perspective? objectivity? Or was it a particular interest in your development?

- If Ana's email arrived in your inbox, how would you respond?

Action Plan

Action 1: Who to approach

Step 1: What is the sphere or setting in which you want to be operating, or are operating?

You may consider completing the following audit:

Professional:		Clinical Specialism:	
AHP		developmental language	
speech and language therapy profession		speech sounds	
healthcare professions		dysphagia	
independent practice		neurology	
academic		emotional and mental health	
research		sensory impairment	
		dementia	
Settings:		emotional and mental health	
public health		sensory impairment	
education		learning disability	
health and social care/public sector		acquired neurological/brain injury	
higher education		special education needs and disability	
research institution			
hospital		**Non-clinical specialism:**	
community		leadership	
early years		governance	
justice		quality	
special education needs and disability		workforce development	
		practice education	
Qualities, skills, attributes		patient involvement/ participation	
		project management	
		leadership	
		governance	

Summary – My "Mentor Specification":

I am seeking a mentor with experience and/or insight into the following areas:

1

2

3

4

Step 2: Having specified the key areas your future mentor will have experience in, like Ana, you will need to consider who to approach. To open your thinking beyond your immediate network, consider:

	Who do I know with the above experience?	*Who do I know of (by reputation)?*	*Who could introduce me to someone in their network?*	*Where else could I look or ask?*
What have I identified in my Mentor Specification (above)?	Already within my network	Social media Publications Podcasts	Friends, colleagues, managers, peers My local network	RCSLT hub RCSLT clinical excellence network RCSLT national office Regional coaching/ mentoring database
1				
2				
3				
4				
5				
6				

Action 2: Approaching a Mentor

What do I need to share with them about myself?	
My profession and career stage	
My dilemma (try composing this as a question.)	
My "ask" – what is the first thing I am asking them to consider?	
How am I going to make this approach?	

Action 3: Preparing for the First Meeting with a Mentor

1. Getting to know one another	What is important for me to share with the mentor?
	What is important for me so that I am sure that this is a person I could trust enough to share my situation with? (some key words about how it will feel)
	What is important for me to understand about the mentor?
2. Decision	We will need to agree whether to progress with mentoring after this initial meeting.
3. Practicalities	What preferences/suggestions do I need to ask the mentor about:
	Face-to-face or remote?
	If face-to-face – preferred place?
	Best times of day/day of the week?
	Length of session. This might be at least an hour, depending on the mentor's preference.
	Is any preparation expected?
	"Contracting" – will there be an exchange of expectations?
	Any information in advance of meetings?

Making the most of my mentoring:	
How will I come to each session fully prepared?	
In what ways will I demonstrate that I am engaged in the session?	
How do I feel about being challenged?	
Do I need to discuss this with the mentor?	
What is my preferred reflective practice?	
Which reflective model will I use (or my own)?	
Where will I record my reflections?	
How will I protect time for reflection after each session?	
How will I identify and complete follow-up actions?	
In what meaningful ways will I show my appreciation to my mentor?	

Further Reading

Chapter 3, "How Can I Be an Effective Client?", in Mary Connor and Julia Pokora's *Coaching and Mentoring at Work* (2007).

References

Blanchard, K. and Diaz-Ortiz, C. (2017) *One Minute Mentoring*. London: Thorson's.

Buning, M. and Buning, S. (2019) *Beyond Supervised Learning: A Multi-perspective Approach to Outpatient Physical Therapy Mentoring*. Augusta, GA: Taylor and Francis.

Coutts, K. A. (2019) Community service speech and language therapists practising in adult dysphagia: Is the healthcare system failing them? *South African Journal of Communication Disorders*, 66 (1), 1–5.

Driscoll, J. (2007) Supported reflective learning: The essence of clinical supervision? In *Practising Clinical Supervision: A Reflective Approach for Healthcare Professionals* (2nd edition). London: Bailliere Tindall. https://shop.elsevier.com/books/practising-clinical-supervision/driscoll/978-0-7020-3247-9

Gibbs, G. (1988) *Learning by Doing: A Guide to Teaching and Learning Methods.* Oxford: Further Education University, Oxford Polytechnic.

Joined Up Careers Derbyshire. Unlocking opportunities in your career. Available from: https://ahpcareers.co.uk/ [accessed on 9/8/2023].

Kline, N. (1998) *Time to Think: Listening to Ignite the Human Mind.* London: Cassell.

Kolb, D. A. (1984) *Experiential Learning: Experience as the Source of Learning and Development.* Englewood Cliffs, NJ: Prentice-Hall.

Moss, W. L., Clem, B. and Wilson, K. (2012) Using technology to mentor aspiring LSLS professionals. *Volta Review*, 112 (3), 329–343.

Pedrick, C. (2021) *Simplifying Coaching.* London: McGraw Hill.

Peltier, B. (2010) *The Psychology of Executive Coaching – Theory and Application.* New York: Taylor and Francis.

Rogers, C. (1951) *Client–Centered Therapy: Its Current Practice, Implications and Theory.* Boston: Houghton Mifflin.

Volkmer, A., Cartwright, J., Ruggero, L., Beales, A., Gallée, J., Grasso, S., Henry, M., Jokel, R., Kindell, J., Khayum, R., Pozzebon, M., Rochon, E., Taylor-Rubin, C., Townsend, R., Walker, F., Beeke, S. and Hersh, D. (2022) Principles and philosophies for speech and language therapists working with people with primary progressive aphasia: An international expert consensus. *Disability & Rehabilitation*, 45 (6), 1–16.

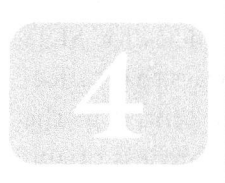

Becoming a Mentor

Introduction

In this chapter, we will explore the skills that are needed for mentors to be impactful, providing a space for the mentee to focus on their goals, as well as challenging the mentee's thinking.

Mentoring and the Speech and Language Therapist's Skillset

In mentoring, the communication skills of one professional have a transformative influence on the other.

The basic skills needed by mentors are core within the skillset of speech and language therapists (SLTs). While some may want to enhance their professional skills through training and reflection, mentoring is a positive way for any SLT to build connections, develop others, and enhance their own skills.

SLTs are experts in communication, and we use our communication skills to transform the lives of people with communication and/or eating, drinking, and swallowing difficulties. Mentoring is a conversation (or a series of conversations) in which the goals of one individual are the focus for the other. SLTs are not alone in this. Any professional who aims to facilitate a transformative effect on another through interaction should be capable of mentoring with impact. As a one-to-one talk-based intervention, is there any need for an experienced SLT to undergo any further training?

DOI: 10.4324/9781003386827-5

Firstly, we should turn to the Health and Care Professions Council (HCPC) Standards of Proficiency that provide the boundaries of our professional practice (HCPC, 2014) and the competencies for SLTs regarding communication. The standards set out the ways that "effective and appropriate verbal and non-verbal skills" are central to the scope of our practice as professionals, as well as an awareness of and ability to use and move between different means of communication. These apply to our work with service users, and also to all of our professional interactions (see Appendix 4.2).

Our training and competencies are set out by the professional body the Royal College of Speech and Language Therapists (RCSLT, 2021) in the guidance that underpins the pre-registration SLT curriculum. The graduate capabilities are the baseline of professional skill. Capabilities of the whole SLT profession, under the headings "communication" and "lifelong learning", intersect when we are considering mentoring (see Appendix 4.1).

The Mentor's Skillset

The key skills of a mentor are:

- listening
- questioning
- building the relationship
- maintaining focus
- supporting learning

No speech and language therapist will read this list and believe that any of the skills are beyond their professional and clinical competence. The list of communication competencies is already core to our work with people with communication and swallowing needs.

In addition, we could add a sixth skill: "advising" or "informing". However, after careful consideration, I have chosen to omit this one.

We mentor from a position of expertise, and at times it will be helpful to the mentee for us to offer ideas, suggestions, and learning from our own experience. But these should be offered only after the person we are coaching has exhausted their own resources. The reason for such a cautious approach is underpinned by neuroscience. Being given advice switches off the person's capacity to learn. We perceive the advice giver as more empowered than we are, as a social threat, and the fight-flight-freeze response is triggered. Hence, we avoid giving advice (Rolfe, 2020, 51). As mentoring is a "learning conversation", we will want to support the individual's ability to learn for themselves, before making helpful suggestions. Of course, equally it would be wrong to withhold information that could be helpful. Pedrick (2021) suggests that we can "change hats with consent". For example: "I wonder if it might be useful for me to share something from my own work?" or "Would it be ok for me to offer a suggestion?" This preserves the autonomy of the learner.

Listening

Clutterbuck (2023) lists five levels of listening: from "waiting to speak" and "listening to disagree" through "listening to understand" to "listening to help the individual understand" and "listening without intent". We can feel that we are really listening well while we are actually "listening to …". Only when we listen without another intention are our minds quiet enough to hear what the speaker is really saying. Our brains can process 500 words per minute. The average speaker produces only 125 words per minute, so listeners have available capacity to listen to ourselves listening (Parsloe and Leedham, 2000) and notice where other intentions might creep in. Be kind to yourself: our active minds are constantly on the lookout for connections with our own experience, with reminders of tasks we need to do, with ideas to benefit the speaker, and being aware of unrelated things in the room. Notice what your mind is doing as you try to listen, and gently refocus on the speaker each time you become aware of a parallel thought stream starting up. "Active listening" rather than peripheral or apparent listening (Parsloe and Leedham, 2000) is "trying to understand not only what is being said but how and why it is being said". As it turns out, active listening requires not only some effort, but also a quiet mind.

Questioning

Questions are the second tool of the mentor. Beyond the mentee's stream of consciousness, questions enable the mentor to "dig deeper" (Pedrick, 2021). Rolfe (2020) offers a mantra for mentoring: "Ask before you tell; listen before you speak". Rolfe proposes that asking questions increases the person's self-awareness, and citing Tasha Eurich (2008), that the evidence that self-awareness is associated with improvements in job satisfaction, progression, and effective leadership.

Writers describe the skill of the mentor's questioning in different ways.

> **For structuring the mentoring session**: Rolfe (2020) summarises the basic questions (however they are expressed) in a session as: "Where are you now?", "Where do you want to be?", "How do you get there?", and "How are you doing now?"

> **Purposes of questioning**: Parsloe and Leedham (2000) describe how mentors use different types of question for the purposes of "awareness raising", "reflection", "justifying", "probing", and "checking".

> **Good mentoring questions**: these are "personal", "resonant", "acute/incisive", "reverberant", "innocent", and "explicit" (Clutterbuck, 2023).

Building the Relationship

We started off in Chapter 1 by identifying that mentoring is a special relationship, and that rapport and the mentor's interest in the person are key. The relationship is focused on the learning, or transformation, of the person being mentored, and in Chapter 3 we considered the mentor's distinct personal motivations. Trust is fundamental in all relationships. In mentoring relationships, trust is earned, or develops, when the mentor and the mentee each demonstrate their adherence to professional values such as confidentiality, integrity, disclosure, understanding, and ongoing review (Starr, 2014). We might pause here and compare the value set of the mentor with the Code of Conduct, Performance and Ethics Standard 2: "be able to practise within the legal and ethical boundaries of their profession" (HCPC, 2014), and note the congruence for us as HCPC registrants.

Starr (2014) likens the mentoring relationship to that of a travelling companion. Her analogy reminded me of Carlos, a walking guide. In 2015 I completed the final 100-kilometre section of the Camino de Santiago di Compostela in Northern Spain. Carlos ensured that my two travelling companions and I reached our daily destinations, as well as the ultimate goal of arriving in the city of Santiago on Day 5. On some sections, Carlos walked with us, chatting to us and learning about our motivations and whether they were physical, spiritual, or cultural. He was interested to understand what motivated us to endure some discomfort and fatigue. He also disclosed something of himself in these conversations and we got to know him and his own vulnerabilities. At other times, he would walk ahead. I remember one day, the longest stretch, when he stood on the brow of a hill and looked back. When we caught up with him, he said we would stop for lunch earlier than planned. This was very welcome news, and I wondered how he knew that we were struggling, what it was that he saw when he looked back. He said: "I see the pace you are walking, and the way you walk, and that you perhaps don't smile back at me, and I know you are tired and hungry". This conversation came back to me as I thought about mentors as travelling companions. Like a mentor, Carlos was more experienced. He knew the route ahead as well as the way we'd come – where the cafes were, the terrain to cross – and he was learning about his walking companions. He'd learned to notice changes in our physical appearance and behaviour that provided clues as to our internal comfort. He had wisdom about the wildlife and the hostelries, and about how to look after blisters! But importantly, he was a living guide who walked with us, rather than a guidebook or audio tour. Mentoring, like being a guide, is a relationship rather than a "self-help" product.

Connor and Pokora (2007) identify the hallmarks of a mentoring, or learning, relationship:

- firstly, after Rogers (1961, 50), "the outer conditions of trustworthiness" – punctuality, confidentiality, and consistency

- secondly, congruence, or genuineness – we sometimes refer to this as "walking the talk"

- thirdly, respect – Rogers' "unconditional positive regard" that underpins all client-centred interactions (Rogers, 1961)

- finally, empathy – the attempt to walk in the other's shoes

Maintaining Focus

Like Carlos, my walking guide, the mentor's role is to ensure we stay on track. When I have someone to take that role, I am free to think, to notice, to dream – without having to worry about getting lost or not arriving on time. The mentor, similarly, keeps one eye on the clock and the other on the person's goals – both their "dilemma" and the question they are focusing on today.

I recommend Claire Pedrick's work (2021) here for her principles of "rightsizing" the question the mentee is seeking to answer. She observes that the "person with the perceived power controls the time", and that managing the time is part of the mentor's role. Her approach "reduces the question to the right size for the time available". In an hour, it is unlikely that Ana's mentor will be able to help her find the answer to "What is my next career move?" or "How can I be happier at work?", but instead "How can I decide what my career options might be?" is right-sized for an hour with a mentor. It focuses on identifying her next steps, her actions, rather than finding a solution in the session. For the mentor, setting out with an achievable task will increase our confidence from the outset.

Starr (2014) highlights removal of "roadblocks and barriers" as part of the way that mentors maintain the focus of the relationship. For example, if my mentee lacks a technical skill, introducing them to a programme of learning may be appropriate. If they would benefit from talking with someone in my network for a specific insight, an introduction is helpful. If their lack of self-awareness limits their aspirations, a psychometric tool may help them to develop their understanding. Rachael supported my learning a few years ago by introducing me to a tool that enhanced my understanding of my own strengths. At the time, I was rather bruised by unsupportive and insensitive feedback. Her recommended tool helped me to identify the "sweet spot" where my interests, strengths, and talents converged, and to review whether I was in the right role at this point in my career.

The mentor shows restraint from offering unsolicited advice, but may identify a barrier to learning. We may suggest something to help the mentee by using our knowledge and relating it to the mentee's dilemma. I see this as distinct (albeit it a nuanced distinction) from offering "should do" and "ought to" types of advice.

Supporting Learning

Mentoring aims for transformation, or growth at least. In this, it is focused on positive future possibilities. The "holy grail" of learning is a new insight. Insights occur through reflection, through reading, through discussion, in silence, but less often in formal learning events like lectures. The mentor will notice when the mentee has a new insight. This may be an obvious "Aha!" or lightbulb moment when suddenly everything becomes much clearer. In my experience, insight-gaining moments often present as the mentee becoming quiet and looking away from the mentor. At those points, my role is to watch and listen, and wait for them to share the new insight, but certainly not to interrupt. A mentor needs to be comfortable with silence and patient to learn what the new revelation might be. Insights could be viewed as the "outcome measure" of a mentoring session. If there is no new insight, there is no learning. If we give the mentee a few moments to summarise what the insights of a session have been, they may be able to distil these. Otherwise, this may occur during their follow-up reflection time. Some of us process new learning more slowly than others.

If insights are the desired outcome of a learning event, then actions are the goal of a transformational conversation. What actions can the mentee commit themselves to? Their summary at the close of the session will draw their focus back to the world beyond the mentoring relationship, and their own responsibility to use their learning for the change they desire. The mentor will notice whether they are recording these actions. Some mentors will expect an update at the next session. Others will see the decision to follow up as the responsibility of the mentee.

Kim's Story (Part 1)

Kim has been approached by Ana, a speech and language therapist who is in her early career, but who is recovering from an incident and seeking a move. Kim is the allied health professions (AHP) lead in a neighbouring area, and also an SLT by professional background. She's been looking for closer links with her own profession since she moved into her current role. Kim is considering Ana's request, and grapples with the term "mentor".

Having agreed to a first meeting, she reflects on this initial encounter. She prefers to use Gibbs' Reflective Learning Cycle (1988) to structure her thinking.

Description: What Happened?

Ana emailed me last month and asked for a "mentoring conversation". She works in a different system, but approached me as a fellow SLT. It turns out there had been an incident that she's trying to put behind her. She has had some counselling through wellbeing support for this.

I was keen to be helpful, but doubted that I have what she's looking for. We met today to discuss what she needs and whether there are any ways that I could help. She summarises her starting point as being at a career crossroads. She's decided to stay in the speech and language therapy profession, but wants to know what her other options are, beyond adult acute inpatients. We ran through some possible options: a lecturer role, another clinical field or a different setting, promotion to a team lead role, or research.

She is really interested in research, and had not believed it was a career option unless you worked in a university.

Feelings: What Were You Thinking and Feeling?

Initially, I was put off by the term "mentoring". Having never met Ana before, I didn't grasp how she could see me as a mentor. I realise that I thought mentors grew out of an ongoing relationship, and hadn't considered that you could just pick one. I almost passed over her request, feeling that I was too busy with people in my own system. Something about her manner made me curious and decided to offer a one-off session – at least so that I could suggest someone more experienced and competent for her to approach.

At the same time, I felt very flattered, because it suggests that my profile as an SLT in a leadership role is known beyond this system. We are a small profession, but I felt I'd "disappeared" within the AHP world and maybe my SLT roots weren't visible within the profession now.

During the session, I felt a lot more comfortable. She reminds me a bit of myself at that stage. She doesn't come from a background where there are loads of role models of healthcare professionals in her family, and having hit her main stumbling block, she was stuck as to where to go next. I sensed that she had overcome a great deal to not have left the profession altogether and found an easier path. In someone of her age, this shows a lot of resilience and commitment, and I'd like to support her if she thinks I can.

Evaluation: What Was Good and Bad about the Experience?

I warmed to Ana as soon as we met. She was respectful of what I have achieved and mindful of other pressures on my time. She came very well prepared, knowing what she wanted, and wrote lots of notes to follow up later. There were points when the conversation seemed to dry up and I thought I'd been too challenging. One of my faults may be that I can be too direct, and

I thought maybe I'd made her uncomfortable. It's been a while since I managed junior therapists, and I wonder if this style can come across as confrontational. I restrained myself from filling the silence a couple of times, and then noticed how Ana came back with something that had occurred to her for the first time. She really seemed to be using the time with me to look at her situation from a new angle.

What I was least comfortable with was Ana's belief that I can guide her into a new career path. The responsibility of leading her in that way makes me a little anxious. I don't know the department that she works in or what her real opportunities are. I felt ill-equipped to be advising or "mentoring" her in that way. Research careers are precarious, and she doesn't have a partner who has a stable job; at the moment, Ana's employment is their main source of income, and her clinical skills are likely to provide them both with more job security.

I also felt wary that Ana has had a traumatic experience at work. I am not part of the system she works in, and I did wonder whether her own managers would view the events in the same way that Ana described them to me. Obviously, this was a confidential conversation, and I would not dream of checking that out. Whatever has happened, Ana is seeking the way forward, and has clearly taken responsibility for her recovery from the harm caused by the incident, as well as thoughtfully looking for someone to help her.

Analysis: What Sense Can You Make of This Situation?

While I felt uncomfortable with the "mentoring" idea, I know I tend to adopt a bit of "imposter syndrome" with new opportunities, and this only lasts as long as I sit and think about it. I've learned to grasp new opportunities with both hands and invariably find I can do better than I expected. If this was a first experience of mentoring, I may have something to offer Ana. She certainly did a lot of thinking and wrote a lot of notes. She said she'd email me back to let me know what she concludes, and if she does (or doesn't!) will be interesting re the actual impact of our session.

I related to her enough to really care how she goes forward. She is short of people to approach – all of the senior professionals in her life have a vested interest one way or another in her staying where she is. Having made a risky move myself out of speech and language therapy and into my current role – taking the secondment rather than staying where I was, I'm perhaps in a good position to support her. I've also had some knockbacks in my time, including times when I thought of giving up and doing something easier instead. I remember my old boss meeting me for a coffee after she'd retired and her being instrumental to some decisions which proved to be good ones. Maybe she was being a bit of a mentor too?

Conclusion: What Else Could You Have Done?

I could have done a bit of research of my own before answering Ana's email, finding out what she might mean by "mentoring". I didn't ask whether the others she'd emailed had responded or not. I don't think she needs more than one mentor for this particular challenge. A quick search has thrown up lots of definitions and examples which help me see this as something that I could have embraced more positively from the start. I'm interested in how much structure to provide in a mentoring session, and whether I should have done more preparation to think of questions to ask Ana. It felt like an exploratory chat. However, just listening and telling Ana what I noticed seemed to help her. I was also able to come up with some actions for Ana to take to find people better equipped to help her find out about research opportunities and training, beyond my knowledge base. So I conclude that the hour and a half we spent together was perhaps more productive for her than I'd have guessed.

Action Plan: If It Arose Again, What Would You Do?

I would certainly like to see Ana again. We left that open, and I'm not sure whether I'll hear from her again. I can see that the time I've spent with her is valuable professional activity for my continuing professional development (CPD). It's made me wonder where AHPs in my own system go for advice and support. I know there is an NHS database of coaches and mentors. I have decided to investigate that – maybe to find someone who could support my own development. I've not yet found a way to stay in touch with the speech and language therapy profession, with physio and occupational therapy taking up most of my time in this role. I will also read more about what good mentoring looks like to see what gaps there are in my own skill set, in case I'm asked again – or in case there is something missing in our system to help the careers of our own AHPs.

Plan:

– wait for Ana to get back in touch
– find out what mentoring opportunities exist in our system – approach the coaching lead
– explore reading/podcasts about mentoring
– file the hours and this reflection in my CPD log

Recap

- mentoring skills are based on the same communication and professional skills that are foundational in speech and language therapy

- the key ingredients of mentoring are:

    - listening

    - questioning

    - building the relationship

- maintaining focus
- supporting learning

  and only a judicious seasoning of information and guidance

- there is a rich variety of resources and books for speech and language therapists to engage with to enhance their mentoring skills

☁ Reflection Prompts

You may find it helpful to pause now to reflect on and note the following:

- Consider the ways in which SLTs use their communication skills to effect transformation on one another's learning.

- Thinking of the "Wise Owls" in your own career (see the section "Reflect" in Chapter 3) whose guidance and time resulted in you taking successful steps forward, what skills do you now recognise that encouraged you, resourced you, signposted you, and resulted in your talent being spotted?

- Which people have you been taking an interest in?

- How does the term "mentoring" fit in with what you're providing?

- How does the term "mentor" fit with your future aspirations?

- What sort of mentoring role might you develop to support someone following their own career journey?

- If you were to observe a good mentoring session, for what percentage of time would you expect the mentor to be speaking? And within that speaking time, what proportion of utterances would you expect to be questions rather than statements?

- What mentoring skills do you think are your strengths? And which need further refinement?

- Who else could provide you with a different perspective on your strengths and development opportunities?

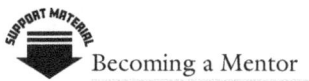

- What behaviours will engender trust in my mentee, to convey trustworthiness, genuineness, respect, and empathy in our mentoring relationship?

- In your clinical work, what is in your tool kit? In which ways are you equipped as a therapist, and could you transfer those skills to mentoring someone?

- Think about the ways you facilitate transformations in:

  - the communication skills of a service user/ client

  - the way a parent/carer relates to your service user/client

  - the way you support a new understanding in colleagues and other professionals

  - clinical supervision sessions

  - leadership appraisals of your team members

  Pick whichever scenario you believe you have the most skill in.

- In what ways are mentoring skills different from clinical skills?

- In what ways would applying mentoring skills described in this chapter enhance your clinical and professional practice?

Action Plan

- What skills do I already have?

- What qualities would I want to develop?

- How might I promote this?

- What could I say to let people know the mentoring door is open to them?

Consider your skill set in relation to the six skills below. Award a total of five points to each skill, dividing them between strengths and development opportunities (for example, if you think you are very skilled at offering advice appropriately, you might give it 5 under strength and 0 under development opportunity).

Mentor Skills	My Strengths	My Development Opportunity
Listening		
Questioning		
Relationship building		
Maintaining focus		
Supporting learning		
Offering advice		

My key mentoring skills are (highest scores under strengths):

These are the foundation of being a great mentor.

My focus for enhancing my mentoring skill set will be (highest scores under development opportunities):

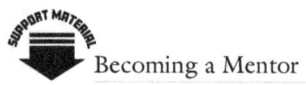
These form the basis of my Mentoring Development Plan.

You may want to write some SMART (Specific, Measurable, Achievable, Realistic, Timed) objectives around these development opportunities as the start of your Development Plan:

Development Goals:	Specific	Measurable	Achievable	Realistic	Timed
1					
2					
3					
4					
5					

Preparing Powerful Questions

Imagine that Ana is coming to see you as one of her "Wise Owls". What are some of the ways you will explore what her next steps are? Write down some questions that you might ask to open up the dialogue and to support her learning:

Questions for Ana:

Now think of someone who looks to you as a more experienced or expert person, and sometimes seeks your advice. Instead of advice, what questions might help them to explore their own development?

> **Questions:**

Developing Coaching Skills

- What is coaching?

- How does it work?

- How could you have a go at practising coaching?

- How can you refine your skills?

- How can you access more training/reading?

- Will you use coaching skills in mentoring or become a coach?

 Further Reading

Nancy Kline's *Time to Think: Listening to Ignite the Human Mind* (1998).
Claire Pedrick's *Simplifying Coaching* (2021).
Ann Rolfe's *Mentoring Mindset, Skills and Tools* (2020).
Julie Starr's *The Mentoring Manual* (2014).

Appendix 4.1: RCSLT Curriculum Guidance

The RCSLT's five core capabilities (RCSLT, 2021) are communication, partnerships, leadership, and lifelong learning, research and evidence-based practice, and professional autonomy and accountability:

> *crucially, SLTs themselves demonstrate adaptability, self-awareness and sensitivity in their own interactions with service users and with members of their teams and other agencies.*

2.1 Communication

Key graduate capabilities:

1. *Demonstrates highly effective and sensitive communication skills in all contexts (SOP 8.1)*
2. *Applies knowledge and skills to transform communication abilities of individuals, groups and communities*
3. *Uses communication skills effectively to negotiate, mediate and influence others*

2.3 Leadership and lifelong learning

Key graduate capabilities:

1. *Demonstrates commitment to, and takes responsibility for, lifelong learning and development of own speech and language therapy practice, and commitment to their role as part of the wider speech and language therapy profession.*
2. *Continually seeks to develop their practice with guidance through reflection and self-evaluation*
3. *Demonstrates critical reflection, resilience, resourcefulness and emotional intelligence*
4. *Demonstrates knowledge of the political, social and cultural contexts within which SLTs work*

5. *Demonstrates commitment and engagement to the role as part of the wider speech and language therapy workforce*
6. *Contributes to the development of the speech and language therapy knowledge and practice of others*
7. *Demonstrates adaptability to changes in speech and language therapy practice and practice environments*
8. *Contributes effectively to innovation and change within area of practice*

Speech and language therapy learners are embarking on a lifelong learning journey, enhancing their unique skillset to enable them to become confident at engaging with new ideas, to build resilience even in challenging times, and to pave the way for others to do the same.

Appendix 4.2: HCPC Standards of Proficiency for Speech and Language Therapists (2014):

8.1 be able to demonstrate effective and appropriate verbal and non-verbal skills in communicating information, advice, instruction and professional opinion to service users, their relatives and carers, colleagues and others.

8.4 be able to select, move between and use appropriate forms of verbal and non-verbal communication with service users and others.

8.5 be aware of the characteristics and consequences of verbal and non-verbal communication and how this can be affected by factors such as age, culture, ethnicity, gender, socio-economic status and spiritual or religious beliefs.

References

Clutterbuck, D. (2023) *Coaching and Mentoring a Journey through the Models, Theories, Frameworks and Narratives of David Clutterbuck*. New York: Routledge.

Connor, M. and Pokora, J. (2007) *Coaching and Mentoring at Work – Developing Effective Practice*. Maidenhead: Open University Press.

Eurich, T. (2008) What self-awareness really is (and how to cultivate it). *Harvard Business Review.*

Gibbs, G. (1988) *Learning by Doing: A Guide to Teaching and Learning Methods.* Oxford: Further Education University, Oxford Polytechnic.

HCPC (2014) Standards of proficiency for speech and language therapists. Available from: https://www.hcpc-uk.org/standards/standards-of-profi ciency/speech-and-language-therapists/ [accessed on 21/08/2023].

Kline, N. (1998) *Time to Think: Listening to Ignite the Human Mind.* London: Cassell.

Parsloe, E. and Leedham, M. (2000) *Coaching and Mentoring: Practical Techniques for Developing Learning and Performance.* London: Kagan Page.

Pedrick, C. (2021) *Simplifying Coaching.* London: McGraw Hill.

RCSLT (2021) Curriculum guidance for the pre-registration education of speech and language therapists. Available from: https://www.rcslt. org/wp-content/uploads/2020/08/RCSLT-Curriculum-Guidance-March2021.pdf [accessed on 21/08/2023].

Rogers, C. R. (1961) *On Becoming a Person: A Therapist's View of Psychotherapy.* Boston, MA: Houghton Mifflin.

Rolfe, A. (2020) *Mentoring Mindset, Skills, and Tools* (4th edition). South West Rocks, NSW: Mentoring Works.

Starr, J. (2014) *The Mentoring Manual.* Harlow: Pearson Education Limited.

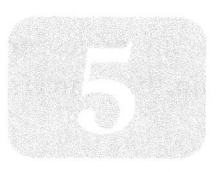

Mentoring for Inclusion

The national outrage and racial unrest, following the killing of George Floyd, turned into a critical inflection point for our professions to address the long-standing lack of racially and linguistically diverse students and professionals in speech-language pathology and audiology.

(Mahendra and Kashinath, 2022, 527).

Introduction

In this chapter, we will focus on the needs of speech and language therapists (SLTs) from groups which are still underrepresented within the speech and language therapy profession. Specifically, this applies to SLTs of colour, LGBTQ+ SLTs, and SLTs with a disability. However, any reader may identify that they represent another demographic within the profession which faces additional barriers in career progression, or which lacks the privileges held by the majority. Furthermore, as a profession, and as a community, we are required to act as allies for one another, challenging the structures and culture that prevent equitable access to any opportunity. This chapter is for everyone: whatever barriers you are facing in your career path, and for the more equitable development of our whole profession – please read on.

I will explore how mentoring could be a helpful tool:

DOI: 10.4324/9781003386827-6

- for diversifying our profession – ensuring that the profession is as varied as the populations we are seeking to serve

- for equality – ensuring that individuals within our profession can enjoy as many opportunities as possible within their careers, regardless of our differences

- for inclusion – ensuring that our profession provides a sense of belonging for all of us

Inequality and Speech and Language Therapy

In 2020, across the world, many of us were reminded of the reality of injustice, firstly by the unequal impact of Covid-19, and then by the killing of George Floyd. The global Black Lives Matter movement brought the reality of institutional racism in society to the attention of those in power once again.

Our profession within the UK started to hear the voices of speech and language therapy practitioners. The RCSLT undertook an investigation of its own governance and published a report called *Toward a More Diverse Board* authored by Kiki Maurey (2021). The report highlighted how the RCSLT was perceived by its members. The professional body was viewed as both "exclusive" and "elitist". During the period when I served on the board, including two years as Chair, a programme of improvements was set out. These included enhanced recruitment and development opportunities to enable more diverse leadership and governance of the RCSLT, and to remove some of the barriers that prevent members from aspiring to and achieving board membership.

As a predominantly white and female profession, privilege is shared inequitably; yet even for those of us who have enjoyed access to education and career development, a glass ceiling still exists at the most senior levels. NHS board positions are still prioritised for doctors and nurses over allied health professionals (AHPs). More broadly, the profession is developed in only a handful of countries: mainly English-speaking and based in the "global North". In a world of inequity, might mentoring be a source of encouragement and career planning for any of us?

Potential opportunities to support further inclusivity across the profession are still numerous, and this focus is ripe for further development.

There is a growing argument for the development of "reverse" or "reciprocal" mentoring. These approaches can provide new opportunities for mentoring to address the inequalities embedded in the communities and institutions in which we operate, and within our own profession. These approaches are of interest to both those providing and those seeking mentoring.

Reverse Mentoring

In reverse mentoring, a "less senior" person is paired with a senior manager within the same organisation to share the person's story, perceptions, and perspective. This enables the more senior leader to be more effective in their role, having gained an enhanced understanding of the other's experience and of their own privilege.

Back in 1999 in a large corporation (General Electric), 500 managers were mentored by younger employees to enhance their understanding of the internet (Greengard, 2002). The skills and lived experience of one person (the expert) in a relationship with another (the novice) was used to enhance the organisation as a whole. This fits our working definition of mentoring. What was different (the "reverse" nature) was that the mentor in this case was younger and less senior than the mentee.

In the new century, the approach started to gain value as a slow growth in society's awareness of institutional privilege (usually in favour of older, white, male employees). Reverse mentoring was adopted by other organisations within their diversity, equality, and inclusion strategies. The approach was applied to a wide range of corporations, enabling people in senior positions to learn from the perspectives of colleagues from underrepresented groups (people of colour, people of faith, women, LGBTQ+) as well as any younger and more junior employees. These "mentors", drawing from their own lived experience, are ideally equipped to mentor their leaders. In return for contributing to the development of the mentee, the "mentor" (the less senior colleague) benefits from the ideas and guidance of the more senior "mentee". Patrice Gordon's (2022) excellent book on this topic describes the changes she led within Virgin Atlantic and emphasises the importance of reverse mentoring as part of an organisational strategy for inclusivity, rather than a stand-alone programme. Such initiatives have also been introduced across NHS organisations and are recognised as an indicator of good practice – for example, Raza and Onyesoh (2020).

A study by Raju (2022) explored the potential of reverse mentoring of consultant physicians by their junior medical colleagues, with the aim of reducing attrition from clinical training programmes by the mentors, and of making improvements in clinical leadership and patient safety by the consultants (the mentees). This programme was designed to enhance the more traditional mentoring model provided within the professional body, the Royal College of Physicians.

Proponents of reverse mentoring emphasise the importance of an adequate framework of support and training to ensure that the mentors can feel safe in speaking honestly to their seniors, and to ensure that mentees are equipped to translate their learning into organisational improvements. Although the rapport or chemistry is still important, these relationships are more likely to be organised by a third party within the organisation, such as the diversity, equality, and inclusivity lead. Alternatively, a senior leader may ask for an introduction to a colleague who has lived experience of what the leader has identified as a blind spot.

Working as an Allied Health Professions' leader in the NHS, I sought an introduction to colleagues of colour from my own profession. In one-off conversations, they talked to me about their career journeys and their challenges and achievements. Making little of some of these challenges, they focused instead on the support they received which had enabled them to arrive in their current roles. I was impacted by the grace they demonstrated while relating some of the obstacles that their white peers had not encountered, for example in completing their pre-registration training or holding on to a registered SLT role. I was struck by the limited progress they had been able to make, despite clear dedication to the profession and their great sense of fulfilment in the roles and teams they now belonged to. Up to this point, I had read and heard about discrimination in my profession, but these conversations came about purely because I asked whether SLTs from an ethnic background differing from my own would be happy to talk to me to enhance my own awareness. I remain very grateful for their time and honesty. I doubt they benefited from the conversation, but my own leadership was enhanced by their generosity. These conversations were not part of a formal reverse mentoring programme and were not supported by training for either the SLT or me. However, the power of curiosity and an open mind – and the willingness to listen and to learn from a person with lived experience – provided me with new insight.

Mentoring for Inclusivity and Diversity

Maybe the risk of the reverse mentoring programme is that the needs of the senior leaders are the focus. Indirectly, through a range of measures aimed at improving inclusivity, the mentors will benefit, but their contribution may be an altruistic contribution to the organisation. So there remains an opportunity for more traditional mentoring (whereby a less senior colleague is mentored by someone more senior).

Some students in all continents are disadvantaged in our predominantly white, female profession. Mahendra and Kashinath's (2022) study (in the context of the US) provided an enhanced student experience for students of communication sciences and disorders who identified as BIPOC (black, indigenous, and people of colour). The aim was to ensure diversity within the student population through enhanced recruitment and retention, to enable the profession to become as diverse as the populations it seeks to serve. Between 2012 and 2017, a training and mentoring programme was introduced at a California state university which included peer and professional mentoring alongside other supports tailored for academic success.

It is well-known that mentoring relationships provide critical, career-long, personal, and professional opportunities. Such relationships are particularly important for underrepresented students and future practitioners who often lack access to informal or formal mentoring networks or to information deemed essential for professional success in healthcare careers.

(Mahendra and Kashinath, 2022, 530)

In their study, peer mentors were paired with students who were newer to the programme, for academic and informal support. Small groups of students were also assigned to "professional mentors" – i.e., practising clinicians. There was a significant improvement in the participants' completion rates for their degrees: "Our findings reveal that BIPOC, and underrepresented students benefitted greatly from regular, structured mentoring and the high-impact nature of research and community engagement projects" (534). The paper also cites Freeman et al. (2016) and Toretsky et al. (2018), whose findings show how minority students in healthcare lack formal or informal mentoring opportunities.

The Mahendra and Kashinath programme was developed in California, where the state population is diverse. In another study, by Girolamo and Ghali (2021) at the University of Kansas, in what they describe as a "white" state, a range of student-led initiatives to reduce the attrition of students from racial or ethnic minority backgrounds from communication science and disorders programmes was developed. Girolamo and Ghali studied the impact of the initiatives, including a multiple mentor model whereby students were trained to be mentored. The study concluded that finding a mentor was reliant on personal connections people from minoritised backgrounds may not have had. Here, maybe, lies a partnership opportunity for universities and employers within our profession that could benefit the profession and its future members and beneficiaries.

George Floyd isn't a "wake up call". The same alarm has been ringing since 1619 – y'all just keep hitting snooze.

(Maurey, 2021, quoting a placard at a Black Lives
Matter demonstration)

International Context

As the profession evolves in the international context, with more countries developing their own speech and language therapists, global opportunities for inclusion across the world will emerge. A study by Atherton et al. (2017) examined the experiences of the first university-educated SLTs in Vietnam. Interviews with these "pioneer" professionals revealed that mentoring support from international colleagues was critical to their emerging practice.

An initiative led by the International Association of Communication Sciences and Disorders (IALP) and the Tavistock Trust provided international mentoring partnerships between SLTs supporting people with aphasia. Feedback from SLTs working in low- or middle-income countries:

> *highlighted the richness of their cultural learning, the value of reciprocal learning, an increased understanding of the challenges experienced by speech and language therapists in under-served countries, and of the importance of mentoring in professional development and in supporting practice with people with aphasia.*
>
> (IALP, 2021)

A similar collaboration, this time between the IALP and Transforming Faces (a Canadian registered charity supporting people with cleft palate and their families), provided international mentoring partnerships.

These informal relationships are supported by international associations and by alliances of SLTs with specific clinical interests. Their early evaluation highlighted benefits, not just for the mentees from under-served countries, but also for the mentors, who gained cultural learning (IALP, 2021).

Conclusion: Reciprocal Mentoring

Through this book, we have reached an understanding that mentoring is not only an altruistic exercise by an experienced and generous individual. As well as that genuine motivation to invest in a less-experienced person, the mentor learns and develops their own insights and skill sets. While reverse (or "upward") mentoring is set to turn the traditional senior–junior or older–younger dyad on its head for the purposes of enhancing inclusivity, the mentor will always gain something from the relationship. Whether we are studying the mentoring of a junior colleague by a senior leader, of a white male leader by a black female employee, or an SLT working in Vietnam by an SLT working in Australia, the mentor gains from the relationship alongside the mentee. The term reciprocal mentoring works well. Whether we are looking at pairs within an organisation, across sectors, or across continents, mentoring has the potential to benefit everyone.

For these reasons, I prefer the term reciprocal mentoring. At this point, we could review our original working definition, and consider whether it covers the variations on mentoring this chapter has described:

Mentoring is a relationship in which one person (with experience in something) invests in the development of another, with altruistic motivation.

In the context of a profession or an organisation where we set out to foster inclusivity, perhaps there is an opportunity to extend this definition and include Patrice Gordon's term: **"building belonging"**.

👤 Kim's Story (Part 2)

Kim is facing a dilemma of her own. Since she first met Ana, she has been challenged about her attitudes to some of her colleagues from different backgrounds. She is reflecting that she has her own blind spots. At an equalities training session, she became more aware of her own privilege, and she painfully acknowledges to herself that she doesn't always understand, or dare to ask, more about some of the people she works with, who feel that she doesn't necessarily understand the barriers that they face at work. As a conscientious leader, she realises that she can either choose to continue, or she can find a safe place to express her curiosity and acknowledge her ignorance, in the interests of becoming a better leader.

Kim wonders if Ana can help. She recognises that Ana's background and lived experiences are very different from her own. Ana has been honest and authentic about herself and doesn't show hesitation in describing the challenges and barriers she faces in her career journey. When Ana asked for mentoring, Kim initially felt like an imposter, partly because she herself has so much to learn from Ana. The term "mentor" didn't sit easily with her.

After several attempts to draft an email to Ana, Kim sends this message:

Hi Ana,

Firstly, I hope you are well, and that the ambitious "to do" list you drew up after our meeting last month is not proving too daunting. Remember I'm here for another conversation whenever the time is right for you.

My reason for reaching out today is a different one. I've found some dilemmas of my own, and I'm wondering if you would be willing to help me.

My own background is different from yours, and I realise that you have faced – and continue to face – challenges that I have little experience of. To be a better leader of all the AHPs, I would like to learn more. I wonder if you would consider mentoring me. Maybe a starting conversation could explore this further? I realise that you are under no obligation at all to do this – and my offer to you to continue to support your development stands, whatever you feel about this request.

Thank you so much for considering it.

Best wishes,

Kim

Ana replies with a tentative but positive response, and a further meeting is set up.

After this meeting, Kim updates her reflective journal:

Description: What Happened?

Ana agreed to meet me to share her experiences. These related to being "different" within her profession and within her workplace. She was tentative at first, but when she realised that I am keen to learn, and that I already see her as an expert in her own life, just as she sees me as an expert in AHP careers, she loosened up. I asked her if she would feel comfortable to tell me a bit about her life so far – particularly the barriers she had to overcome to get into her professional training, to identify role models, and to find ways to be "her authentic self" at work. She talked then for about 20 minutes. I just listened.

Feelings: What Were You Thinking and Feeling?

Initially, I was nervous. I felt like I was prying and that I was maybe asking her to expose feelings – vulnerabilities – that she would not want to share with me. It felt really intrusive. However, as she got warmed up, she started to expand beyond the facts, and into her own feelings. At points, she became teary. I felt a little uncomfortable about this, but checked if she was happy to continue. She was emphatic that she wanted to, if I didn't mind the emotion. That was all fine with me. It showed we were getting to the heart of her experience. I also felt honoured that she could trust me with this. She shared so much about her struggles as a student, when she felt different from her peers, and that her practice educators weren't always aware of how hard she was working to get the same progress as other students. I wondered if she had role models that she followed, and was shocked that she didn't meet another SLT with the same background until she had been working for a couple of years, and at that stage a staff network was set up. I'd never considered how hard it is for people to make time from clinical work to attend those networks, and I'm quite ashamed that I had sometimes seen them as a bit of a skive from work. I now realise that the feeling of belonging

98

and of connection is vital. I've always found myself surrounded by colleagues whose lives have followed similar paths to my own. I've not considered how "othered" some people might feel among a homogenous workforce like AHP (and especially like SLT). It was a real eye-opener. I started to feel very unworthy and uncomfortable, and I almost asked Ana to end the session. Then I noticed how energised she was becoming and that she was having some new insights of her own – it wasn't clear who was mentoring whom, we were both learning with each minute that passed.

There was one very long silence. I'm not great with these, and this doubled my own discomfort, but I managed to restrain myself from interjecting. Ana was thinking, and then told me something that really impacted me. Thankfully, I gave her the permission to think well, and to share something profound, once she had gathered her thoughts.

Evaluation: What Was Good and Bad about the Experience?

I felt very uncomfortable all the way through the session. While that seems a bad thing, I realise that there is no learning in the comfort zone! Ana made my learning as safe as she could. I asked some questions, and she was both gentle and firm with me. I learned that I have been using some expressions that weren't helpful. She put me right, and I have noted what terms she prefers – but also that this is how Ana wants to refer to herself at this point, not how everyone does.

At one point, I got the role of mentee really wrong – I told Ana "what she should do". She very firmly reminded me that in this conversation she is the expert, and that I haven't walked in her shoes yet. I immediately apologised, and she accepted very graciously ("I'm used to it!") and continued. I settled back into "learner" mode and let go of my management ego for a bit.

I was also concerned that I had underestimated the other barriers that Ana has had to deal with. I didn't know that she also has a disability, although she wasn't even planning to share this with me. She did so when it became clear that her identity is multifaceted and that she can't be put into a simple pigeonhole. She wanted to tell me more about this condition because she knows we often overlook intersectionality, and it's an easy (lazy) error when we are considering diversity.

On the positive side, I've learnt so much. Not only about Ana's story, but I am learning not to make generalisations, not to avoid asking people for their own preferences, terminology, or to tell me what I can do to help. I have felt scared of getting it wrong in the past – of using the wrong term, not being correct, and of causing offence. None of these is a bad thing – but the fact that they stopped me getting close to the person, asking them what matters to them and inviting them to put me right, closed me off to learning. No wonder my colleagues have been a little critical of my approach. I feel a load (a fear) has been lifted – all I must do is ask, and learn.

I also feel really motivated to continue down this line of enquiry, now that the door is open, there are so many more opportunities to explore.

Analysis: What Sense Can You Make of This Situation?

That there's nothing wrong with ignorance. We all start off with our own set of experiences. But that refusing to learn more is just arrogant, and in my position of leadership, I am duty bound to continually learn – not just about policy, or clinical issues, but also about the people I lead. They are so much more diverse than I had acknowledged. Ana is my first teacher in this, and she has been generous – and courageous.

Also on the plus side – Ana said she feels more comfortable about reaching out to me next time, because she feels like there is "give and take" rather than her "taking up my *precious* time".

Painfully, I'm wondering what it's really like to be on the receiving end of me. I realise that I'm too ready to rest on my expert position and think I'm paid to know it all. I know very little about many things, but the good news is there are kind teachers all around who are the real experts – like Ana. I'm considering where else I can take my learning (e.g., executive coaching). This learning goes way beyond the context of my conversation with Ana and is likely to be a long journey.

Conclusion: What Else Could You Have Done?

I could have asked Ana more pertinent questions when we first met. I would have been a better mentor if I had acknowledged that she and I have different backgrounds, and that her whole identity contributes not only to the dilemma she was facing, but also to the way she approaches new opportunities. It might only have taken an extra ten minutes in our initial conversation to have found out a bit more. Not that what she took away was limited by my oversight, but I lost out on my own learning. I wonder if we needed to do the switch from Kim the Mentor to Ana the Mentor. If I had opened up the conversation more curiously and more bravely (and sensitively), I might have learnt more from Ana as we went along.

Action Plan: If It Arose Again, What Would You Do?

Having found that there is a mentor database that I have joined, I will update my profile to say, "I'm learning more about my own bias and privilege, and I'm committing to use my position for the benefit of increased inclusivity in the workplace." If there was another opportunity, I'd like to explore with Ana what she feels about the concept of "allyship" which is being promoted in our organisation, and which (I confess now) I was a little sceptical about.

Plan

- Write to thank Ana – she has been courageous, generous, candid. She has invested some time in me and offered to help again in future.

- Check that she is OK, having shared a lot with me, and see if there is anything I can do as follow-up.
- Reiterate that I am also here for her and remain committed to her development.
- Be really specific about what I have learnt from her – including better ways of using language and overcoming some of my previous ignorance (more discomfort!).
- Reiterate that I can guarantee her confidentiality, privacy, an open door, interruption-free conversations in the future, plus any signposting to safeguard her as she helps me learn.
- Tell my personal assistant that communications from Ana are to come direct to me and not be filtered to anyone else.
- Give myself a day or two and then list the learnings – and the actions that arise for me from this rich conversation.

Ana emails Kim:

Hi Kim,

Today was brilliant – not easy, but I could see you learned something from our chat, and I also had some new thoughts and realisations about myself. I've never seen myself as a leader, and that certainly isn't my career path. But I do see that if I can influence a shift in some of your thinking, our relationship will have a much wider impact than I could ever have on my own. Thank you for asking me. I'm looking forward to our next session (I'll bring some of my own questions and let you know how my own voyage of discovery is going).

Best wishes,

Ana

🔔 Recap

- the world is inequitable, and power and privilege sit unequally with some groups

- the speech and language therapy profession is not as diverse as the populations we seek to serve. Some SLTs face barriers that others (the majority) don't

- those with more power and privilege can be allies and share opportunities with those who are currently disadvantaged within society and within institutions

- if we recognise that "expertise" in mentoring includes our different lived experiences, mentoring becomes reciprocal – and not hierarchical

- there is a particular value when SLTs (and students) from communities (countries) that are still underrepresented and disadvantaged in the established profession access mentoring

- this work has only started, and there is plenty to do

- everyone can learn something from one another – win–win!

💭 Reflection Prompts

You may find it helpful to pause now to reflect on, and note:

- In what ways am I like the majority of SLTs in the profession?

- In what ways do I differ? Have these differences ever impaired my sense of belonging or identity as an SLT?

- How easy was it to find role models like me during my career, especially early on?

- Are there others in my network about whom I have limited understanding? What could I do to address this?

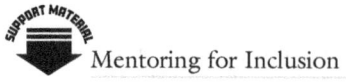

- What opportunities might there be to open new conversations to help my own learning?

- How could I use my own lived experience to support the learning of someone else? Am I ready to share if I'm asked?

Action Plan

Next Steps

Thinking about:

Finding out:

Asking about:

Doing:

Further Reading

Patrice Gordon's *Reverse Mentoring: Removing Barriers and Building Belonging in the Workplace* (2022).

References

Atherton, M., Davidson, B. and McAllister, L. (2017) Exploring the emerging profession of speech-language pathology in Vietnam through pioneering eyes. *International Journal of Speech-Language Pathology*, 19 (2), 109–120.

Freeman, B. K., Landry, A., Trevino, R., Grande, D. and Shea, J. A. (2016) Understanding the leaky pipeline: Perceived barriers to pursuing a career in medicine or dentistry among underrepresented-in-medicine undergraduate students. *Academic Medicine*, 91 (7), 987–993.

Girolamo, T. M. and Ghali, S. (2021) Developing, implementing, and learning from a student-led initiative to support minority students in communication sciences and disorders. *Perspectives of the ASHA Special Interest Groups*, 6 (4), 768–777.

Gordon, P. (2022) *Reverse Mentoring: Removing Barriers and Building Belonging in the Workplace*. New York, NY: Hachette Go.

Greengard, S. (2002) Moving forward with reverse mentoring. *Workforce*, 81, 15.

IALP (2021) Supporting speech and language therapists working in low income countries working with individuals with aphasia first report in Enderby, P (2023) Private correspondence [email] sent to M. *Heritage*, 12 September.

Mahendra, N. and Kashinath, S. (2022) Mentoring underrepresented students in speech-language pathology: Effects of didactic training, leadership development, and research engagement. *American Journal of Speech-Language Pathology*, 31, 527–538.

Raju, S. A., Ching, H., Jalal, M., Lau, M., Rej, A., Tai, F. W. D., Tun, G., Hopper, A. D., McAlindon, M. E., Sidhu, R., Thoufeeq, M. and Sanders, D. S. (2022) Does reverse mentoring work in the NHS: A feasibility study of clinicians in practice. *BMJ Open*, 12 (11), 1–6. https://bmjopen.bmj.com/content/bmjopen/12/11/e062361.full.pdf

Raza, A. and Onyesoh, K. (2020) Reverse mentoring for senior NHS leaders: A new type of relationship. *Future Healthcare Journal*, 7 (1) (February), 94–96.

Maurey, K. (2021) *Toward a More Diverse Board*. London: RCSLT. Available from: https://www.rcslt.org/wp-content/uploads/2022/05/RCSLT-Board-Report-March-2021-Kiki-Maurey.pdf [accessed on 28/09/2023].

Toretsky, C., Mutha, S. and Coffman, J. (2018) *Breaking Barriers for Underrepresented Minorities in the Health Professions*. University of California San Francisco: Healthforce Center.

A Vision for Collaborative Mentoring

Introduction

In this chapter, I will make a proposal for how speech and language therapists (SLTs) could work as a professional community to ensure that each member has access to the benefits of mentoring, both as a mentor and for their own development.

The original concept was suggested in a short article in the *RCSLT Bulletin* (Heritage, 2021). In this article, I described how SLTs have the skills required to provide mentoring. I outlined the idea that if every member of the profession mentored one other SLT, the whole profession would have significantly more capacity for support, guidance, and continuing professional development (CPD). This concept became the basis for this book.

Looking back on the main points of the book – the benefits of mentoring, the existing evidence base for enhanced career progression, and the close match with the SLT's skill set – leads me to conclude that mentoring is an underutilised resource in the profession's tool kit.

Before returning to that vision, I will offer a possible explanation for how the profession has managed so well without adopting mentoring more widely. A helpful insight comes from the work of Kram and Isabella (1985). The authors of this paper were, at the time, professors of organisational behaviour in the US. While their work is almost 40 years old, it still has relevance for our profession today. Citing Levinson et al. (1978), Clawson (1979), Kram (1985), and Phillips

DOI: 10.4324/9781003386827-7

(1977) to outline how younger adults benefit from mentoring in their early careers and describe the importance of a range of work-based relationships that contribute to professional development, they went on to study the impact of peer relationships.

Peer Relationships

Kram and Isabella highlight the availability of peers relative to mentors. The absence of hierarchy in the peer relationship "might make it easier to achieve communication, mutual support, and collaboration" (Kram and Isabella, 1985, 112). While earlier studies had focused on men, this one ensured equal numbers of female and male participants. This is important when applying their research to our own profession, with 98% of members being female. The study examined the role of peer relationships across the ages and stages of the career lifespan. Their findings suggest that:

> *peer relationships offer an important alternative to conventional mentoring relationships by providing a range of developmental supports for personal and professional growth at each career stage.*
> (Kram and Isabella, 1985, 116)

What is striking to an SLT is the rich resource of peer relationships that provide support, guidance, and encouragement between peers. From my own observations and experience, peer friendships formed at university, through subsequent work roles, and postgraduate study programmes are maintained for many years, and often throughout the whole career. Friendships within the profession are treasured, and importantly continue to provide many of the same benefits as mentoring. Maybe SLTs have less need for formal mentors than other professionals because of the rich network of peers that we build throughout our working lives? Certainly, I can track many of my own friendships 40 years back to my bachelor's degree programme, my first SLT role as a graduate, my new service manager peers, and my AHP Lead counterparts. The periods of time when we are training – both at pre-registration and for postgraduate qualifications – seem to consolidate particularly close friendships between work peers, some of which are sustained far beyond the study programme. The people we learn alongside and the people we work with seem to become particularly significant in our development.

Kram and Isabella (1985) identified career progression and professional confidence as the benefits of peer relationships. They described the characteristics of the relationship that contributed to these outcomes: shared values, emotional support, personal feedback, and mutuality (i.e., the relationship is reciprocal, not hierarchical). Significantly, peer relationships commonly bridge different stages of a career: "some peer relationships seen in our study began in early career and continued through late career lasting as long as 20 or 30 years" (Kram and Isabella, 1985, 118).

The study also identified stages of peer relationships along a continuum: from "information peer", characterised by exchange of knowledge, to "collegial peer", with increased levels of trust and disclosure, to "special peer". Special peers resemble close friendships, covering home life as well as work, developing over years, and withstanding transitions. As well as longevity, peer relationships differ from mentoring relationships in that a mentor has additional experience relative to the mentee, while peers are more likely to offer a two-way exchange of support. Their conclusion is that mentors are most important in early careers, while peers may sustain the need for a long-term supportive relationship throughout the career life span.

Figure 1.2 in Chapter 1 showed the territory covered by mentoring and other similar but distinct supportive relationships. When considering where to place "peer" along the objectivity or context-specificity continuum, I concluded that "peer" occupied the same space as "mentor" – at the intersection of the two. A peer may be either involved or objective, working in the same or a different context. This reinforces the overlap between the function of mentors and the function of peers.

In Chapter 5, we identified an additional purpose for mentoring in our profession, that of inclusivity, which has much more focus in the twenty-first century than it did in the 1980s. A definition of "peers" could be "people like me". We have noted that the reliance on peers and personal networks can exclude those who are already marginalised in our profession. Having a network of peers is part of the privilege of belonging. Again, we see how mentoring can play a supportive role for those who are first entering the profession (or aspiring to), or who are on the margins of the profession, until they have built their own peer networks.

Furthermore, I suggest that mentoring can provide additional "scaffolding" to those, like Ana, who are transitioning from one career path to another. Here, our existing peer relationships may lack the expertise and insight needed. Maybe our need for mentoring ends at the point when we have established a peer network in the new stage of our career.

A Vision

This book has outlined the importance, potential, and opportunities for mentoring in the speech and language therapy profession. For the uptake of mentoring to move forward, we will need a common understanding of what mentoring is, what it is not, what it can achieve, and what behaviours are likely to underpin effective mentoring. Mentoring could be integral to our communities of practice:

- clinical excellence networks
- regional hubs
- pre-registration study programmes
- postgraduate study programmes
- leadership networks
- research networks
- the global SLT/SLP community

We can be more conscious, more curious, and more intentional within these communities by asking "where are my blind spots?" "Who is on the margins of this group?" "Who is not yet included?" Formal training in how to mentor and how to be mentored would be advantageous, but not essential. The exercises within this book will help to resource both the mentor and the mentee. Learning these skills as a pre-registration student will lay down essential leadership skills and will foster the discipline of developing colleagues and peers, as well as our service users. We can continue to value and nurture those "special peer" relationships described above.

So how could the profession sustain its own mentoring needs? Mentors need to be able to identify themselves and what they can offer. Mentees need a clear idea of what they are looking for from a mentor. A platform is needed to connect one with the other. This can be as simple as mentors publicising what they have experience and expertise in, and mentees identifying their best match. Doing this online could be relatively simple, whether at a local level or nationally within a specialism, or even internationally.

It is my view that mentoring has a positive impact on inclusivity, professional development, and workforce retention, widening participation and improving wellbeing. Each of these is a critical priority for our profession if we are to optimise our impact on communities we seek to serve.

🔔 Recap

- mentors provide valuable contributions to the development of:
  - career entry
  - transition from pre-registration to newly qualified practitioner
  - people who are marginalised within the profession
  - career crossroad and transition points
  - early leadership development

- peer relationships develop during a career. These mutual relationships provide many of the benefits of mentoring

- "special peers" are the most longstanding and trusting of peer relationships, and may last the entire extent of a career

💭 Reflection Prompts

You may find it helpful to pause now to reflect on, and note:

- Who do you consider to be your peers in relation to your work?

- With which of these peers do you exchange information?

- With which peers do you have sufficient trust to share more personal details?

- Who are your "special peers" – those that have lasted more than one career change, or if you are just setting out on your SLT career, which of your peers might at some point achieve this status?

- In what ways do you invest in these important peer relationships to ensure that they will stand the test of time and provide ongoing mentoring-type value in your life?

- What else do you need at this point that your peers cannot provide and that you may look for in a mentoring relationship?

- What else might your peers be unable to fulfil in the future that a future mentor may contribute?

- What are your opportunities in your networks or in your leadership roles to develop mentoring relationships between members?

References

Clawson, J. G. (1979) *Superior-Subordinate Relationships for Managerial Development*. Unpublished doctoral dissertation. Harvard Business School, Boston.

Heritage, M. (2021) *A Mutually Beneficial Relationship*. London: Redactive. RCSLT Bulletin, No. 827.

Kram, K. E. (1985) *Mentoring at Work: Developmental Relationships in Organizational Life.* Glenview, IL and New York: Knopf.

Kram, K. E. and Isabella, L. A. (1985) Mentoring alternatives: The role of peer relationships in career development. *Academy of Management Journal,* 28 (1), 110–132.

Levinson, D. J., Darrow, C. N., Klein, E. B., Levinson, M. A. and McKee, B. (1978) *Seasons of a Man's Life.* New York: Knopf.

Phillips, L. L. (1977) *Mentors and Proteges.* New York: Arbor House.

Index

Page numbers in **bold** refer to Figures.